From Freud's Consulting Room

Also by Judith M. Hughes

To the Maginot Line: The Politics of French Military Preparation in the 1920's (1971)

Emotion and High Politics: Personal Relations at the Summit in Late Nineteenth-Century Britain and Germany (1983)

Reshaping the Psychoanalytic Domain: The Work of Melanie Klein, W. R. D. Fairbairn, and D. W. Winnicott (1989)

JUDITH M. HUGHES

From Freud's Consulting Room

The Unconscious in a Scientific Age

Harvard University Press

Cambridge, Massachusetts, and London, England   1994

Library of Congress Cataloging-in-Publication Data

Hughes, Judith M.
   From Freud's consulting room : the unconscious in a
   scientific age / Judith M. Hughes.
      p.   cm.
   Includes bibliographical references and index.
   ISBN 0-674-32452-8 (alk. paper)
   1. Freud, Sigmund, 1856–1939.   2. Subconsciousness
      —History.   3. Psychoanalysis—History.
   4. Clinical psychology—History.
I. Title.
BF109.F74H845   1994
150.19'52'092—dc20   93-47172
CIP

Designed by Gwen Frankfeldt

Photograph of Freud's consulting room on p. xi
courtesy of Edmund Engelman

For Allan D. Rosenblatt and Melford E. Spiro

Acknowledgments

When I am working on a book, I like to talk—and talk—about it. And over the years I have found a number of ready listeners, who have allowed me to try out ideas that were tentative or fragmentary and who have responded with queries and suggestions. Though they may not immediately recognize how they made a contribution to the final product, I do, and would like to thank the following: Roy G. D'Andrade, Reva P. Greenburg, Patricia W. Kitcher, Donald L. Kripke, George Mandler, Michael Meranze, Robert S. Westman, and Robert M. Young. When the book was just about finished, Aïda D. Donald, editor-in-chief of Harvard University Press, gave it a careful reading and strong endorsement, and then Anita Safran did a discriminating and sensitive job of copy-editing.

In London I incurred debts of gratitude to two directors of the Freud Museum, Richard Wells and Erica Davies, who gladly put at my disposal the Freud-Ferenczi correspondence. In La Jolla, I enjoyed and profited from the Psychoanalytic Interdisciplinary Seminar sponsored by the Department of Psychiatry at the University of California, San Diego. Very early on I presented to its members what I thought was an outline of a possible project. They good-humoredly but firmly told me that I had offered two possibilities, not one, that I had better make a choice, and also indicated their own preference. On this last point they were unanimous. Though the end result may bear only a slight resemblance to their recommendation, I am grateful for both the matter and the manner of the advice given. Roughly halfway through the writing, I became a clinical associate at the San Diego Psychoanalytic Institute. The last chapter benefited most from this new affiliation, and I want to thank my colleagues for helping me read clinical material as if I were behind rather than simply on the couch.

Once again the person who has borne the brunt of my talk has been my husband, Stuart. He has listened as I have struggled aloud to formulate lines of argument and to decide upon organizational tactics and strategy. He has read more than one version and has offered editorial suggestions each time round. And once again he has been patient and forbearing.

.   .   .

I am grateful to Sigmund Freud Copyrights, The Institute of Psycho-Analysis, and The Hogarth Press for their kind permission to quote from *The Standard Edition of the Complete Psychological Works of Sigmund Freud,* translated and edited by James Strachey. Permission has been granted by Basic Books, a division of HarperCollins Publishers, Inc., to quote excerpts from "Freud's Psycho-Analytic Method" (*The Collected Papers of Sigmund Freud,* Volume 1), "Fragments of Analysis of a Case of Hysteria" (Volume 3), "Analysis of a Phobia in a Five-Year-Old Boy" (Volume 3), and "Notes upon a Case of Obsessional Neurosis" (Volume 3); authorized translation under the supervision of Alix and James Strachey. Published by Basic Books, Inc., by arrangement with The Hogarth Press, Ltd., and the Institute of Psycho-Analysis, London.

Contents

Contents

From Freud's Consulting Room

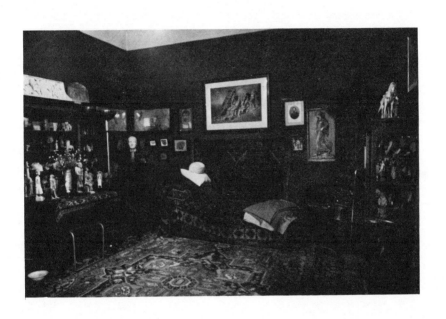

Introduction

Over the past twenty-odd years a shift has taken place in writing the history of psychoanalysis. What had generally been considered the private preserve of the analytic profession, despite poaching on the part of intellectual historians and critics, literary and social, has become a topic for historians of science.[1] It is under the rubric history of science, broadly conceived, that my study falls.

Past and present historians of psychoanalysis, their divergent views about its founder and the nature of what he founded notwithstanding, have emphasized the interdisciplinary quality of Freud's project: its dependence on and/or transformation of ideas from a wide range of disciplines. And along with this emphasis has come a concentration on theory and metatheory at the expense of clinical practice and the clinical setting.

To these remarks Henri Ellenberger stands as a partial exception. He set an interdisciplinary agenda, and a rewarding one; yet he also located "Freud's incontestable innovation" in a "new mode of dealing with the unconscious, that is, the psychoanalytic situation."[2] Here he alluded to another and complementary agenda—to trace the emergence of psychoanalysis as a discipline in its own right—and implied that Freud's clinical material would figure as central to it. I have taken that suggestion to heart.

In reading William James's *Principles of Psychology* (1890) I was struck by the philosophical riddles he felt obliged to tackle, chief among them the relation between mind and body and how the mind could know things in a surrounding physical world. Here were long-standing conundrums that handicapped him in his attempt to establish a naturalistic science of psychology. I could not help wondering whether such concerns might have represented formidable obstacles for Freud as well.

But Freud was no James. Unlike James, he was disinclined to tackle metaphysical and epistemological problems in the abstract. As I see it, he did tackle them nonetheless—in his clinical practice. For when he encountered hysterical patients, that is, patients suffering from somatic symptoms for which he could find no organic cause, he could not duck the mind-body problem. He reached an impasse. He found a more fruitful approach when, to account for his patients' difficulties, he turned to sexuality and reconceptualized it as psychosexuality. In similar fashion, when in his clinical practice he tried to sort out the value of memories, how the mind appraised the external world and stored that appraisal, he came up against epistemological riddles. A standoff ensued. Once again psychosexuality, this time applied to the external world, more particularly to mothers and fathers, proved the fruitful approach. Hence it occurred to me that by organizing the clinical material along philosophical axes I might be able to trace how Freud gave a new (might one say revolutionary?) twist to traditional problems, and how in this unfamiliar guise they became familiar as central preoccupations within psychoanalysis.

My study starts with a chapter comparing James and Freud. Both would rank as men of science, but they were very much at odds with one another over the status of an unconscious domain. Three chapters follow, arranged topically rather than chronologically: the first traces how Freud rethought the mind-body problem and included the body as a source of meaning in the unconscious; the second how he rethought the subject-object problem and included the object world again as a source of meaning in the unconscious; the final chapter takes up the therapeutic "conversation" he devised to explore that domain. This organization reflects my general purpose: to depict the emergence of an autonomous discipline dedicated to the exploration of unconscious meaning.

Readers who know their Freud should be forewarned. They should not assume that the "Freud" to whom they have grown accustomed will necessarily be the "Freud" they encounter in these pages. Here the argument is cumulative. I have refrained from forecasting at every turn what lies ahead and instead have coaxed the clinical material into telling a coherent story. In each of that story's sub-plots, I have resisted the temptation to give the dénouement away. My hope is to engage my readers, to induce them to look at the past, in this instance the past of psychoanalysis itself, in a new way.

CHAPTER ONE

Space for Meaning/Intention/Purpose

In close to the last paragraph of *On the Origin of Species* (1859) Charles Darwin penned a purposefully cryptic, purposefully pregnant remark: "Light will be thrown on the origin of man and his history."[1] Who could doubt it? Who could doubt that the *Origin*'s sustained argument for the uniformity of nature would have implications for the study of man? Nothing except the laws of nature—no intentional or intervening Providence—governed the natural order. Those laws included evolution through natural selection; and that order included man. Thanks to changes in both organic and inorganic conditions, a place, an environmental niche, had opened up for this ape-like being. Variation and selection had done the rest.

If a place had opened for man, along with it went a niche for his mind. Or did it? Was brain all that mattered? On this issue Darwin's adherents did not speak with a single voice; among them divergence was the rule. More than a century and a quarter later, that divergence is still with us. The question then as now is not so much philosophical as one of a research agenda—whether or not to take into account what people report about thoughts and feelings.

Freud was determined to listen, more particularly, to his patients. So too was William James. Why bother with James? There is no evidence that Freud read James's work, although he had met the American psychologist and philosopher in 1909 on his one visit to the United States.[2] James, then, cannot rank as an "influence" on Freud. His function is largely representative: he stands for the exploration of the psychological region in a post-Darwinian scientific world; he stands for the farthest limit of such exploration—before Freud.

James himself was explicit in acknowledging the positive impact of what he referred to as the "biological study of human nature. . . . A band of workers full of enthusiasm and confidence in each other," he wrote, in an essay entitled "A Plea for Psychology as a 'Natural Science,'" was "pouring in materials about human nature so copious that the entire working life of a student" might "easily go to keeping abreast of the tide." What subject matter belonged, by right, to the members of this band who wanted to call themselves psychologists? James plumped for "mental state" as "the fundamental datum" of a discipline he hoped would become scientific.[3]

A Focus on Consciousness

Phenomena which suggested mental processes going on outside or on the margins of consciousness represented a continuing intellectual concern throughout James's career.[4] He read about these phenomena and did research on them, and over time their fascination for him became increasingly manifest. Three texts serve as benchmarks: *The Principles of Psychology,* published in 1890; the Lowell Lectures on exceptional mental states, given in 1896; and *The Varieties of Religious Experience,* first delivered as the Gifford Lectures and later published in 1902.

Two contemporary writers influenced James's discussion: Pierre Janet and Frederic W. H. Myers.[5] The French researcher—he was at the very least a philosopher, physician, and psychologist—had published *L'Automatisme psychologique* in 1889, and James reviewed it in an essay entitled "The Hidden Self." The British investigator, a founding member of the Society for Psychical Research, published his work, "The Subliminal Consciousness," in 1892. (James himself served as president of the society in 1894–96.)[6] Janet wrote of primary and secondary personages, of consciousness being split into parts; Myers wrote of the subliminal mind, of that part of the mind which lay below the threshold of normal, waking consciousness. Much of James's own account was shaped with an eye to assessing these competing hypotheses.

Janet and his co-workers had discovered that consciousness in hysterics, the objects par excellence for inquiry and experiment—and also treatment—was very curious indeed: it seemed to come and go. James provided examples. A patient whose whole side was supposed to be without sensation was told to say "yes" whenever he felt a pinch and "no" when he felt none. His eyes were bandaged for good measure. When the anesthetic side was touched, instead of saying nothing, he responded by commenting that he felt nothing. Obviously he would not have replied unless he had felt *something*. Another example, this one of hysterical blindness in the left eye: when a prism was held before the patient's right eye, both eyes being open, she immediately proclaimed that she was seeing double. Again she would not have replied unless her left eye was being used simultaneously with her right. A more complex example was furnished by one of Janet's star patients, Lucie:

> Lucie . . . would awaken in the middle of the night, light her lamp, and proceed furiously with house cleaning. . . . Once when someone holding a lighted lamp followed her and tried to get her attention, Lucie failed to react in any way to the person's voice or gestures. But when her own lamp began to falter, she attended to it immediately. Lucie's anesthesia extended only to those objects to which she elected to pay no attention. When she carried her own lamp, she would attend to no others. Regardless of the number of lamps in the room, she would call it completely dark if hers was unlit.[7]

Janet had also discovered, so James reported, that by "various odd processes" the anesthesias themselves "could be made to disappear more or less completely." Magnets, plates of metal, electrodes of a battery placed against the skin were some of the items endowed with this "peculiar power." Doubly peculiar: when one side was relieved, the anesthesia was often found "to have transferred itself to the opposite side," which until then had been well. Hypnosis or the hypnotic state turned out to be more potent still—so Janet learned in experimenting with Lucie. During one session she lost consciousness and upon reviving was plunged into a trance unlike that which hypnosis usually induced. In the usual sort of hypnotic trance, Lucie's anesthesias were merely diminished; in this deeper trance, they were entirely gone. Lucie, so it seemed, had been transformed into a different person, with different sensibilities, different memories—and a normal one to boot.[8]

Of Janet's cases, the one James found most "deeply suggestive" was that of Marie. The nineteen-year-old girl had come "to the hospital in an almost desperate condition, with monthly convulsive crises, chills, fever, delirium, attacks of terror, etc., lasting for days, together with various shifting anaesthesias and contractures all the time, and a fixed blindness of the left eye." Seven months elapsed without any change in the patient's condition and without Janet doing anything more than a "few hypnotic experiments and a few studies on her anaesthesia." Her despair at last led him to question her more closely about the onset of her symptoms. She could not answer; she could not remember or remembered only indistinctly. Hopeful that in a deeper trance the memories would return, Janet induced such a state. Symptom by symptom he proceeded to track down the experience that had accompanied its first appearance. The hysterical blindness of Marie's left eye, for instance, had its origins in her sixth year, "when she had been forced, in spite of her cries, to sleep in the same bed with another child, the left half of whose face bore a disgusting eruption. The result was an eruption on the same parts of her own face, which came back for several years before it disappeared entirely, and left behind it an anaesthesia of the skin and the blindness of the eye."[9]

The symptoms ranked as commonplace; the cure did not. The "artifice" Janet hit upon consisted in carrying Marie "back in imagination to the earlier dates."

> It proved as easy with her as with many others when entranced, to produce the hallucination that she was again a child, all that was needed being an impressive affirmation to that effect. Accordingly, M. Janet, replacing her in this wise at the age of six, made her go through the bed-scene again, but gave it a different *dénouement*. He made her believe that the horrible child had no eruption and was charming, so that she was finally convinced, and caressed without fear this new object of her imagination.

When awakened, Marie was able to see clearly with her left eye. In similar fashion Janet cured her other symptoms. Five months later, he reported in his book that Marie continued well, had put on weight—indeed showed no trace of hysteria. In the end, she also proved "no longer hypnotizable."[10]

From hysteria James passed on to cases where the division of personality was more obvious, and gaps in consciousness correspondingly wider. Here he could also pass on to a patient of his own: Ansel Bourne, an itinerant Rhode Island preacher. Bourne had myriad hysterical symptoms, but it was as a "case of alternate personality of the 'ambulatory' sort" that James introduced him. He had been "subject to headaches and temporary fits of depression . . . during most of his life, and . . . [had] had a few fits of unconsciousness lasting an hour or less," as well as suffering from "a region of somewhat diminished cutaneous sensibility on the left thigh." Otherwise his health was good—and, more important, his character upright. No one who knew him, James wrote, could doubt the genuineness of his tale.

> On January 17, 1887 he [Ansel Bourne] drew 551 dollars from a bank in Providence with which to pay for a certain lot of land, . . . paid certain bills, and got into a Pawtucket horse-car. . . . He did not return home that day, and nothing was heard from him for two months. . . . On the morning of March 14th, however, at Norristown Pennsylvania, a man calling himself A. J. Brown, who had rented a small shop six weeks previously, stocked it with stationery, confectionary, fruit and small articles, and carried on his quiet trade without seeming to anyone unnatural or eccentric, woke up in a fright and called in the people of the house to tell him where he was. He said his name was Ansel Bourne, that he was entirely ignorant of Norristown, that he knew nothing of shop-keeping, and that the last thing he remembered—it seemed only yesterday—was drawing money from the bank, etc., in Providence.

In June 1890 James persuaded the patient to submit to hypnosis. In a hypnotic trance, James hoped, "Brown" memories would come back and, following his own suggestion, the two personalities might be induced to "run . . . into one." James's skill as a hypnotist proved sufficient to produce Brown's reappearance; his powers of suggestion, however, were not up to the task of bringing about a fusion of Brown and Bourne. In this instance no artifice availed to make the memories continuous: in a waking state Bourne had no knowledge of Brown; in a trance state he remembered only "Brown's" brief existence and nothing of his normal life—not even his wife. "Mr. Bourne's skull," James wrote, apparently contained "two distinct personal selves." He concluded that the case should "be classed as one of spontaneous hypnotic trance, persisting for two months"—with the added peculiarity that "nothing else like it" had occurred in the man's life, and that "no eccentricity of character" had come out.[11]

In the case of Ansel Bourne, the second self bore some resemblance to the primary self—James described the Brown personality as a "rather shrunken, dejected, and amnesic extract of Mr. Bourne himself." In that of Lurancy Vennum, the second self bore no such resemblance—it claimed to be the spirit of "Mary Roff (a neighbor's daughter, who had died in an insane asylum twelve years before)." For the latter, which James regarded "as extreme a case of 'possession'" as one could find, he drew on a published account appropriately entitled *The Watseka Wonder.* Prior to declaring herself Mary Roff, Lurancy, age fourteen, had lived, not exactly quietly, with her family in Watseka, Illinois. She had already manifested numerous hysterical symptoms and fallen into spontaneous trances. Upon making the astounding declaration as to her identity, she insisted upon returning "home," that is, to the Roffs' house. "The Roffs, who pitied her, and who were spiritualists into the bargain, took her in."[12]

> The girl now in her new home, seemed perfectly happy and content, knowing every person and everything that Mary knew when in her original body, twelve to twenty-five years ago, recognizing and calling by name those who were friends and neighbors of the family . . . calling attention to scores, yes, hundreds of incidents that transpired during her [Mary's] natural life. During all the period of her sojourn at Mr. Roff's she had no knowledge of, and did not recognize any of Mr. Vennum's family.[13]

After eight or nine weeks in the Roff household, Lurancy began to return for a few minutes—only occasionally and only partially. After fourteen weeks, the "Lurancy-consciousness came back for good."[14] Mr. Roff reported:

> "She wanted me to take her home, which I did. She called me Mr. Roff, and talked with me as a young girl would, not being acquainted. I asked her how things appeared to her—if they seemed natural. She said it seemed like a dream to her. She met her parents and brothers in a very affectionate manner, hugging and kissing each one in tears of gladness. She clasped her arms around her father's neck a long time, fairly smothering him with kisses."[15]

Eight years later Lurancy was "married and a mother, and in good health. She had apparently outgrown the mediumistic phase of her existence."[16]

What did James make of these strange phenomena? Initially, he seemed ready to adopt Janet's formulation: "splitting up of the mind into separate consciousnesses." The French psychologist, he wrote, had proved "one thing conclusively, namely that *we must never take a person's testimony, however sincere, that he has felt nothing, as proof positive that no feeling has been there.*" The feeling might belong to the "consciousness of a 'secondary personage'" of which the primary one was ignorant. "That the secondary self or selves," co-existed "with the primary one, the trance-personalities with the normal one, during the waking state," he reckoned to be Janet's great discovery. But he was not persuaded that the secondary self was always "a symptom of hysteria." He was not persuaded—as Janet's theory entailed—that the "primary and secondary consciousness added together" could "never exceed the normally total consciousness of the individual."[17] In short, James gave Janet credit for Marie, but found him wanting in the case of Lurancy Vennum, whose two consciousnesses seemed to surpass the Frenchman's prescribed limit.

With such a case, the views of Myers came to the fore. In his lectures on exceptional mental states, James introduced—and it ranked as one of the most important ideas of the series—Myers's notion of supraliminal and subliminal consciousness, that is, an everyday waking state and a consciousness beyond the margin. Myers himself characterized this subliminal reality in terms of a progression:

> At the inferior end, in the first place, it includes much that is too archaic, too rudimentary, to be retained in the supraliminal memory of an organism so advanced as man's. . . . The recollection of processes now performed automatically, and needing no supervision, drops out from the supraliminal memory, but may be in my view retained in the subliminal. . . . In the second place, and at the superior . . . end, the subliminal memory includes an unknown category of impressions which the supraliminal consciousness is incapable of receiving in any direct fashion, and which it must cognize, if at all, in the shape of messages from the subliminal consciousness.[18]

Myers's formulation, James told his audience, worked "better" then Janet's. It was the more inclusive: both the normal and the pathological came within its jurisdiction. It fitted cases covered by "the formula of dissociated personality" as well as ones which suggested "supernormal powers of cognition." At this point James drew back, concluding, "with great diffidence," that the only thing he was "absolutely sure of" was "the extreme complication of the facts."[19]

.　　　.　　　.

In James's view, consciousness, whether split-off or subliminal, still figured as consciousness. He shied away from the assumption that states of mind could be unconscious. What alarmed him was not the notion of unconscious mental states per se, but what he called the "mind-stuff" theory, that is, conceptualizing mind as so much "stuff" or "dust" which grew "by accretion from lesser to greater units."[20] The mind-stuff theorist, James argued, felt "an imperious craving to be allowed to *construct* synthetically the successive mental states" which he described. Unconscious mental states offered endless opportunities to satisfy that craving. They were "the sovereign means for believing what one likes in psychology, and of turning what might become a science into a tumbling ground for whimsies."[21]

Of the so-called proofs for unconscious mental states that James listed, if only to refute them, the tenth and last stood out as being less obviously deficient. It was also the one which rested on evidence most readily grasped, as he put it, by "human beings—with heads on their shoulders":[22]

> There is a great class of experiences in our mental life which may be described as discoveries that a subjective condition which we have been having is really something different from what we had supposed. We suddenly find ourselves bored by a thing we thought we were enjoying well enough; or in love with a person whom we imagined we only liked. Or else we deliberately analyze our motives, and find that at bottom they contain jealousies and cupidities which we little suspected to be there. . . . All these facts, and an enormous number more, seem to prove conclusively that, in addition to the fully conscious way in which any idea may exist in the mind, there is also an unconscious way.

James's response amounted to a curt dismissal:

> There is only one "phase" in which an idea can be, and that is a fully conscious condition. If it is not in that condition, then it is not at all. Something else is, in its place. The something else may be a merely physical brain-process, or it may be another conscious idea.[23]

Freud's "rebuttal"—five years after James's death—was equally trenchant:

> This objection is based on the equation—. . . taken as axiomatic—of what is conscious with what is mental. This equation . . . either . . . begs the question whether everything that is psychical is also necessarily conscious; or else it is a matter of convention, of nomenclature. In this latter case, it is, of course, like any other convention, not open to refutation. The question remains, however, whether the convention is so expedient that we are bound to adopt it.

Freud considered it most inexpedient. To opt for a physical definition of what was unconscious would force one "to abandon the field of psychological research prematurely," to abandon it "without being able to offer . . . any compensation from other fields."[24]

A Focus on the Unconscious

> The concept of the unconscious has long been knocking at the gates of psychology and asking to be let in. Philosophy and literature have often toyed with it, but science could find no use for it. Psycho-analysis has seized upon the concept, has taken it seriously and has given it a fresh content.[25]

Freud wrote these lines in 1938; they were published in 1940, a year after his death. He had initially mentioned the unconscious in print more than four decades earlier, in 1895.[26] Roughly midway between these dates, in 1912 and 1915, he offered thorough accounts of his hypothesis about unconscious mental processes. The first came in response to an invitation from the Society for Psychical Research to contribute to its *Proceedings*. The second figured in a series of highly theoretical essays Freud wrote during the First World War.[27] The first was addressed to an audience largely unfamiliar with his own work, but well acquainted with that of James, Janet, and Myers. The second represented a summing up of his thought, part personal meditation, part legacy to his most faithful followers. Taken together, they made clear what was distinctive about the psychoanalytic concept of an unconscious domain.

In his "Note on the Unconscious in Psycho-Analysis" written (in English) for the London-based Society, Freud distinguished three different notions. The first was descriptive: it was adjectival and nothing more. It connoted all those contents that were not present in the field of consciousness at a given moment. The second notion was that of the dynamic unconscious. Here Freud reminded his audience of experiments demonstrating post-hypnotic suggestion and of the rich symptomatology displayed by hysterical patients. In both the "artificial" world of hypnosis and the "natural" world of hysteria, one found "plenty of . . . facts" showing that the mind was "full of active yet unconscious ideas." A hypnotic subject, for example, having been awakened and seemingly in his "ordinary condition," would be seized "at the prearranged moment" by "the impulse to do such and such a thing," and he would do it "consciously, though not knowing why. . . . Only the conception of the act to be executed . . . emerged into consciousness. All the other ideas associated with this conception—the order, the influence of the physician, the recollection of the hypnotic state, remained unconscious." Similarly, a hysterical woman "executing the jerks and movements constituting her 'fit,'" would not be able to explain what she intended. Analysis, however, would "show that she was acting her part in the dramatic production of some incident in her life, the memory of which was unconsciously active during the attack."[28]

Along with this dynamic conception, Freud introduced a distinction between different kinds of unconscious ideas—between preconscious and unconscious proper. The distinction hinged on admissibility to consciousness: preconscious ideas could pass into consciousness without difficulty, whereas unconscious ideas remained such and seemed "to be cut off from consciousness."[29] In Janet's work, admissibility and inadmissibility to consciousness could not be conceptualized: the division between his primary and secondary personages or consciousnesses was a "kind of natural or brute fact"; it resembled "a fissure in some geologically weak section." At this point Freud had parted company with him.[30] (As for Myers, Freud did not refer to his writings—parapsychology he flirted with, but rarely in public.)[31]

In the final paragraph of his essay, he mentioned a third notion, that of a system unconscious[32]—a notion he elaborated in his 1915 paper. Here he explicated the relations between this and other systems by framing two competing hypotheses: the topographical and the functional. (To indicate that he was using the terms in a systemic sense, he employed the abbreviations Cs. for consciousness, Pcs. for the preconscious, and Ucs. for the unconscious.) Topography, Freud quickly pointed out, had "nothing to do with anatomy"; it referred not "to anatomical localities, but to regions in the mental apparatus," wherever they might be "situated in the body." According to the topographical hypothesis, the transposition of an idea from the Ucs. to the Pcs. (or Cs.) involved "a fresh record" or "a second registration" of the idea in question; that is, alongside the original unconscious record, which continued to exist, a second registration was required in its new psychical locality. According to the functional hypothesis, the transposition of an idea from one system to another consisted in "its abandonment of those characteristics peculiar to the old system and its adoption of those peculiar to the new"—which Freud summed up as a "*functional* change of state."[33]

In order to choose between the two hypotheses, he surveyed clinical evidence derived from his work with hysterics and other neurotic patients. The case of a hysterical girl whose mother had informed him of the homosexual experience which apparently lay behind her daughter's attacks seemed promising. When Freud told the story to the girl, she responded with another attack and promptly forgot the story. He tried again, with the same result: every time he repeated her mother's story, the girl "reacted with an hysterical attack, and . . . forgot the story once more." Finally, to protect herself from further repetition of story and attack, "she simulated feeble-mindedness and a complete loss of memory."[34] Before she sank into that condition, she had had "the same idea in two forms in different places" in her mental apparatus: initially, she had had the unconscious memory of her experience as it had occurred; subsequently, she had had "the conscious memory . . . of the idea," conveyed in what Freud had told her. At first glance, evidence of this sort would seem to indicate that unconscious and conscious ideas were "distinct registrations, topographically separated, of the same content." On closer scrutiny, the difficulties the patient experienced in making a connection between the unconscious memory trace and the conscious thought process suggested that the transition from one system to another involved a functional change of state. At this stage Freud refused to render a verdict.[35]

It was the behavior of schizophrenic patients that helped him come to a decision, or rather, prompted him to bring forward a third hypothesis. A patient of Freud's had retreated from life because of what he perceived to be the condition of the skin on his face. He was certain that he had blackheads and deep holes which were visible to everyone. "At first he worked at these blackheads remorselessly; and it gave him great satisfaction to squeeze them out, because, as he said, something spurted out when he did so. Then he began to think that a deep cavity appeared wherever he had got rid of a blackhead, and he reproached himself most vehemently with having ruined his skin for ever by 'constantly fiddling about with his hand.' Pressing out the content of the blackheads," Freud concluded, was "a substitute for masturbation." The cavity that emerged as the result of his patient's ministrations was in his mind the female genital. "The cynical saying, 'a hole is a hole'," allowed shallow pores in the skin to represent the vagina. The "sameness of words" rather than a "resemblance between the things denoted" accounted for the symbolism in question.[36]

This example pointed to the distinction on which Freud's third hypothesis rested—the distinction between word and thing presentations. Thing presentations were built up out of "the direct memory-images of the thing" or at least out of "remoter memory-traces" derived from direct ones. Word presentations were also built up out of mnemic residues, but in this instance, residues of seeing and particularly of hearing a word. The actual statement of the third hypothesis became a simple next step: the system Ucs. contained the thing presentations; the system Pcs. housed the word presentations; and thing presentations could not become preconscious or conscious until they became linked with mnemic residues of words.[37]

What advantage did this hypothesis have over its rivals? All at once, Freud claimed, it became absolutely plain wherein lay the difference between a preconscious and an unconscious presentation. Neither of the earlier hypotheses had indicated that a preconscious idea differed from an unconscious one in the complexity of its presentation. Only this third hypothesis, which had no specific name attached to it, pointed to the necessity of a dual presentation: for an idea to be preconscious, for a person to make use of it or to think about something, required the linking of two combinations of residues. Without such a linkage the idea remained in the Ucs.[38]

What advantage did the notion of a system unconscious have over that of a dynamic unconscious? In proposing the former Freud was extending the range of the mental once again: latent characterized ideas that were unconscious in a descriptive sense; latent yet active characterized ideas that were unconscious in a dynamic sense; latent yet active but never yet consciously perceived characterized ideas that were unconscious in a systemic sense.

> The content of the Ucs. may be compared with an aboriginal population of the mind. If inherited mental formations exist in the human being—something analogous to instinct in animals—these constitute the nucleus of the Ucs.[39]

(Given the limited capacity of consciousness, a notion such as the system unconscious might suggest itself as an "expedient . . . convention." Whether to ascribe to it "inherited mental formations" would be another matter.) Though Freud was subsequently to revise his model of Cs., Pcs., and Ucs., by then the system unconscious had achieved its goal: it had provided conceptual space for phenomena that, as Freud put it, had "sense," and by sense he understood "meaning, intention," and "purpose."[40]

One final question. Did Freud discard the dynamic unconscious in favor of the systemic? Far from it. The dynamic unconscious, and its companion concept, repression, remained constitutive of the psychoanalytic domain. An original act of repression could account for an idea's exclusion from consciousness; continuing pressure of that sort could account for further and ongoing banishment; but it was only when the repressed returned—when what had been unconscious emerged into consciousness—that it became possible to get a handle on its meaning.[41]

. . .

The schema of word and thing presentations enabled Freud to conceptualize the relation between preconscious and unconscious; it provided leverage when it came to interpreting unconscious contents as well. And Freud had had it at his disposal before his patients started telling him their dreams, and he began to "move the infernal regions."[42]

This schema had already put in two appearances. Freud initially employed it in his 1891 monograph *On Aphasia,* and in so doing he acknowledged his debt to the British neurologist John Hughlings

Jackson.[43] Among possible neurological mentors whom Freud had encountered, whether through their writings or through their teaching, Jackson alone had made the difference between consciousness and unconsciousness hinge on the word. (The word itself, Freud wrote, was a complex presentation "constituted of auditory, visual, and kinaesthetic elements.")[44] He employed the schema next in his "Project for a Scientific Psychology" (1895), his unpublished and aborted speculation on the neurophysiology of mind. How, Freud wondered, could a thought process construed in quantitative terms acquire the quality necessary to become perceptible to consciousness? (Consciousness he conceptualized as "a sense-organ for the perception of psychical qualities"—only by being highly saturated with sensory content could an idea attract consciousness to itself.)[45] He surmised that "*indications of speech-discharge* . . . put thought-processes on a level with perceptual processes"; such indications conferred the requisite sensory content.[46]

In *The Interpretation of Dreams* the linkage between word and thing presentations found a further application: for thing presentations, Freud substituted wishes; for word presentations, residues of the dream-day. Wishes played a double role: they were both mundane and theoretical. A wish could be very mundane indeed. Freud's youngest daughter, aged nineteen months, after an attack of vomiting and consequently a day spent without food, cried out in her sleep: "Anna Fweud, stwawbewwies, wild stwawbewwies, omblet, pudden!" In this case, as was frequently true with children, the wish had not bothered or been obliged to conceal itself. In their theoretical guise wishes played a role, a crucial role, in the mental apparatus. It was a wish derived from "an experience of satisfaction," that is, an impulse aimed at reinstating a once satisfying situation that "set the apparatus in motion." Freud's theory of the dream as "the (disguised) fulfillment of a (suppressed or repressed) wish" was thus bound up with his more general conception of mind.[47]

Where, Freud asked, did wishes that were fulfilled in dreams come from? There were three possibilities: they had been aroused during the day, consciously acknowledged, but left unsatisfied; they had been aroused during the day, but had been repudiated; they had "no connection with daytime life" and became active only at night. These three kinds of wishes could be assigned to different psychical localities: the first belonged to the preconscious; the second had been driven from the preconscious into the unconscious; the third was "altogether incapable of passing beyond the system Ucs."[48]

By the same token, the three kinds of wishes were not of "equal importance for dreams"; they did not possess "equal power to instigate them." A conscious wish or a preconscious one, Freud hypothesized, could instigate a dream only if it succeeded *"in awakening an unconscious wish* . . . and in obtaining *reinforcement from it."*[49] (By unconscious wish he meant a wish belonging to the system Ucs., more particularly one of "infantile origin.")[50] To unconscious wishes he thus granted pride of place. To explicate the alliance formed between preconscious and unconscious wishes, he drew an analogy. A daytime wish could be likened to an entrepreneur who had the idea or initiative for a project but lacked the financial resources to carry it out; he needed a capitalist, and in the case of a dream, the capitalist who provided "the psychical outlay" was "indisputably . . . *a wish from the unconscious."* Variations on the analogy sprang to mind: there might be more than one entrepreneur; there might be more than one capitalist; or the capitalist might himself figure as an entrepreneur also.[51]

Like wishes, "day's residues" were both mundane and theoretical. On the mundane level, Freud was not alone in observing that dreams showed "a clear preference for the impressions of the immediately preceding days," that in every dream it was possible "to find a point of contact with the experience of the previous day," and that an "indifferent impression" invariably contributed to the dream's content.[52] To explicate the function and functioning of a recent, though indifferent, impression, he once again resorted to an analogy, this time to an American dentist. The dentist was forbidden to "set up in practice" unless he could find a "legally qualified medical practitioner to serve as a stalking horse and to act as a 'cover' in the eyes of the law." Just as it was not "the physicians with the largest practices" who formed "alliances of this kind with dentists," so too, Freud continued in a less homely and more theoretical vein, conscious or preconscious ideas that had already attracted considerable attention would "not be chosen as covers for a repressed idea." The freshness of an impression, as well as its unimportance, meant that its associative capacity (which was assumed to be limited) was still available; it might still serve as a node to which the intensity of an unconscious wish could be attached.

19

And its triviality allowed it to escape repression, or rather to escape repression's first cousin, censorship.[53]

To look for the day's residues suggested itself as a logical strategy for beginning a dream's interpretation. It was also frequently the "easiest."[54] But no method guaranteed that an interpretation would be "complete." Did Freud think it practicable to strive for a "complete" interpretation? In 1911, in a short paper entitled "The Handling of Dream-Interpretation in Analysis," he gave an answer by and large in the negative. The consequences, however, he did not regard as irreparable. "In general," he argued, one could "rest assured" that wishful impulses which created "a dream to-day" would "re-appear in other dreams" and possibly in a "more accessible form." It might be asking a great deal of physician as well as patient to "abandon themselves to a guidance" which seemed "accidental!" But only by such an open-ended procedure could wishful impulses be "withdrawn from the domination of the unconscious."[55]

.   .   .

"Human megalomania," Freud wrote, had had to submit to both a biological blow and a psychological one. Of the two, the psychological was the more wounding. Current research, he claimed, sought "to prove to the ego" that it was "not even the master in its own house, but must content itself with scanty information" about what was going on "unconsciously in its mind." And the current researchers who were engaged in the "most forcible" seeking were, of course, psychoanalysts.[56] It was they, and above all Freud himself, who had undertaken to explore the unconscious domain.

CHAPTER TWO

Redefining the Body

Does the body interact with the mind? If so, how? From the seventeenth century on, these questions, and Descartes's dualistic answer to them, had been central to philosophical-psychological discussion. Even when psychologists, in the course of the nineteenth century, slowly came to distinguish themselves from their philosophical forebears, they did not renounce their inheritance of metaphysical worries. Freud himself took that step only gradually—and not fully consciously.

What were his views on the mind-body problem? In his *On Aphasia*, Freud subscribed to John Hughlings Jackson's psycho-physical parellelism, which pictured the psychic as "a dependent concomitant" of the physiological.[1] In his metapsychological paper "The Unconscious," he appeared to back away from that position; in an off-hand fashion he referred to the "insoluble difficulties of psycho-physical parallelism" without pursuing the issue.[2] When one reads through his other psychoanalytic works "looking for pronouncements on . . . the mind-body problem," one "cannot fail to be struck by the way Freud managed to avoid committing himself."[3] It would seem, then, that what he thought about this problem, at least as it has figured in philosophical journals, has not been particularly fruitful.

Still, the metaphysical tradition continued to intrude. How could it do otherwise, once Freud had encountered hysterical patients and decided to introduce the body into the unconscious domain? He did that and rather more than that: he reconceptualized the body so introduced. He then gave a new (revolutionary?) twist to the mind-body problem: it became a matter of bodily experiences endowing the ego (understood as self) with meaning, and in this fashion, as Freud tersely remarked, the ego became "first and foremost a bodily ego."[4]

Psyche and Soma

On July 13, 1883, Freud wrote to his fiancée, Martha Bernays, reporting, as was his wont, on the day's events. It had been the "hottest, most excruciating day of the whole season," and he had been "really almost crazy with exhaustion. . . . Badly in need of refreshment," he had gone to see his friend and mentor Josef Breuer. The first thing Breuer did was to "chase" Freud "into the bathtub," which had a tonic effect. Then the two men had supper in their shirtsleeves and engaged in "a lengthy medical conversation on moral insanity and nervous diseases and strange case histories—. . . [Martha's] friend Bertha Pappenheim also cropped up"—and finally the talk became "rather personal and very intimate."[5]

Freud and Breuer's friendship dated back to at least 1877. Gradually the older man—Breuer was his friend's senior by fourteen years—became one of Freud's financial patrons and professional advisers. Breuer played the latter role with circumspection. His advice took the form of disabusing his junior of illusions, without, however, scotching his enthusiasm. He understood his young friend too well for that. Breuer, Freud wrote his fiancée, told him "he had discovered that hidden under the surface of timidity" there lay "an extremely daring and fearless human being." Freud himself had always thought as much, but he had "never dared tell anyone."[6] Almost a decade later, in 1895, Breuer wrote Wilhelm Fliess, his successor as Freud's confidant-in-chief, that Freud's intellect was "soaring at its highest," and that he could only gaze after him "as a hen at a hawk."[7] By then the hen and the hawk had grown estranged.

Who was Josef Breuer in his own right? In the first instance he was a physiologist of considerable renown. Students of medicine encounter the Hering-Breuer reflex and the Mach-Breuer flow theory of the vestibular apparatus. The former refers to the self-regulating mechanism of breathing controlled by the vagus nerve, the latter to the function played by the semicircular canals in the ear. In 1875, on the strength of this work, Breuer became a Privatdozent at the University of Vienna. Ten years later he resigned his position (an unorthodox move which signaled his recognition that a professorship was out of the question) without, however, abandoning his research interests. In the second instance Breuer was known as an outstanding physician. "Not only did he appear to everyone the clear-sighted informed diagnostician and the cautious but . . . successful therapist; he also showed himself to those physicians who learned from him and who sought his advice to be a serious scholar and thinker who probed deeply into the obscure connection between normal and pathological processes."[8] In the third instance he was a man of cultivation, with a circle of friends and acquaintances extending beyond the field of medicine. Philosophers and writers figured among them, and he himself possessed a rich store of knowledge in art and the humanities. He drew on that store, along with his physiological understanding and his clinical sagacity, in grappling with the case of Bertha Pappenheim, alias Anna O.

Breuer treated Anna O. from late 1880 to mid-1882. "This," as Freud noted in his *Autobiographical Study,* "was at a time when Janet's work still belonged to the future," before Janet had treated Lucie and Marie and hence before Freud—or Breuer for that matter—could have read about these cases. Both men "repeatedly" read about Anna O., that is, "pieces of the [original] case history,"[9] a full copy of which—as well as a follow-up detailing the medications given her to treat a severe facial neuralgia—were recently found at the Sanitorium Bellevue in Kreuzlingen near Konstanz.[10] (She was a patient there from July 12 to October 29, 1882.) Breuer had apparently drafted the original case history when she was admitted; one of the doctors at the sanitorium had composed the follow-up when she was released. (It was not until the late 1880s that she regained her health.) Breuer was once again reading his own account as he put together the chapter he devoted to Anna O. in his and Freud's joint work, *Studies on Hysteria.* The two versions are not identical, but reasons for the discrepancy are not known. The first deals more extensively with the patient's family—a subject which, even after more than a decade, Breuer could not discuss publicly without being indiscreet. The second version alone recounts the fourth period of her illness, the period that Breuer found most illuminating.

When Anna O. fell ill in 1880, she was twenty-one years old. Hers had been the usual upbringing of a daughter of an orthodox and prosperous Viennese Jewish family, that is, one that concentrated on religious training—reading essential biblical texts and learning the appropriate prayers as well as mastering the rules for supervising a Jewish kitchen—and neglected a secular education. She probably stopped attending school at the age of sixteen. Anna herself, according to Breuer's unpublished report, "was not at all religious. . . . In her life religion" served "only as an object of silent struggles and silent opposition." It might have been otherwise with university studies or a useful occupation—had she been given a chance. She had, Breuer noted, "remarkably shrewd powers of reasoning and clear-sighted intuition." He regretted that she had not received "the solid nourishment" her "powerful intellect" required.[11] (A decade and a half later she in fact became a leader in Jewish social work.)

The course of her illness, Breuer wrote, fell into four clearly marked phases: "latent incubation" from mid July to December 1880; "manifest illness" lasting until sometime in the spring of 1881; "a period of persisting somnambulism" which continued until December of that year; and finally a "gradual cessation of the pathological states and symptoms up to June, 1882." Those symptoms were legion. Here is a partial listing:

> Left-sided occipital headache; convergent squint . . . markedly increased by excitement; complaints that the walls of the room seemed to be falling over . . . ; disturbances of vision . . . ; paresis of the muscles of the front of the neck, so that finally the patient could only move her head by pressing it backwards between her raised shoulders and moving her whole back; contracture and anaesthesia of the right upper, and, after a time, of the right lower extremity. . . . Later the same symptom appeared in the left lower extremity and finally in the left arm.[12]

Of crucial concern to Breuer were Anna O.'s peculiar mental states. Even before her illness became manifest, she had been observed "to stop in the middle of a sentence, repeat her last words and after a short pause to go on talking." She had long been accustomed to engage in what she described as her "private theatre"—embellishing her monotonous existence almost continuously with "systematic day-dreaming." This habitual "living through fairy tales in her imagination" passed over "without a break" into *absences.* Though she was not conscious of it, the absences gradually increased. When in November 1880 Breuer was called in to treat a severe cough of Anna's, which he diagnosed as a typical *tussis nervosa,* he recognized at once that he had to deal with "two entirely distinct states of consciousness . . . which alternated very frequently and without warning."[13]

The absences (they "later became organized into a *'double con-science'*")[14] in which Anna hallucinated and was "'naughty'—that is to say, she was abusive, used to throw cushions at people, so far as the contractures at various times allowed, tore buttons off her bedclothes and linen with those of her fingers which she could move and so on"—certainly ranked as a peculiar mental condition. Equally peculiar was the sequence that occurred every afternoon and evening. Anna would first fall into a somnolent state and then into a still deeper sleep. After about an hour of such sleep, she would grow restless and repeat the words "tormenting, tormenting." What was tormenting her? During her daytime absences she had been heard to mutter a few words, hinting at a narrative she was embroidering. If, in the evening, someone reproduced those muttered words—the someone soon became Breuer and Breuer alone—"she at once joined in and began to paint some situation or tell some story." Her tale finished, she would wake up in a calm frame of mind. (Later in the night "she would again become restless, and in the morning, after a couple of hours' sleep, she was visibly involved in some other set of ideas.")[15] If for some reason, such as Breuer not being present, she failed to tell him her story, she also failed to calm down, and the following day she would have to tell him two stories in order to be quieted.

The auto-hypnosis which "remained constant throughout the . . . eighteen months . . . she was under observation" (the sequel is still a mystery) furnished Breuer with insight into what was going on during the absences. In the fourth and final phase of the illness, it furnished him with "insight into the . . . pathogenesis of this case of hysteria" as well. The initial new oddity was a change in the content of her absences. At the start Anna's alternating states of consciousness had "differed from each other in that one (the first) was the normal one and the second alienated"; at the onset of the fourth phase "they differed further in that in the first [state] she lived," like everyone else, "in the winter 1881–2, whereas in the second she lived in the winter 1880–1"; to be exact, she lived through that winter day by day. Her evening sessions now became "heavily burdened": Anna "had to talk off not only her contemporary imaginative products but also the events and 'vexations' of 1881." Strange though this might be, stranger was still to come. A third and crucial "group of separate disturbances" turned up in the evening sessions: "these were the psychical events involved in the period of incubation of the illness between July and December 1880." It was these, Breuer concluded, "that had produced the whole of the hysterical phenomena."[16]

The phenomenon, or symptom, which intrigued Breuer most was Anna's paralyzed right arm. His account of its origin ran as follows. In July 1880, while in the country, Anna's dearly loved father became seriously ill (he died the following April) and she immediately took up the nursing duties. One night, sitting at his bedside, "in a great state of anxiety about the patient, who was in the high fever," Anna "fell into a waking dream and saw a black snake coming towards the sick man from the wall to bite him." (Breuer interpolated that she had previously been frightened by snakes in the field behind the house, and thus had "material for the hallucination.") "She tried to keep the snake off, but it was as though she was paralyzed. Her right arm . . . had gone to sleep and had become anaesthetic and paretic; and when she looked at it the fingers turned into little snakes with death's heads." The whistle of a train blew and broke the spell.

> Next day, in the course of a game, she threw a quoit into some bushes; and when she went to pick it out, a bent branch revived her hallucination of the snake, and simultaneously her right arm became rigidly extended. Thenceforward the same thing invariably occurred whenever the hallucination was recalled by some object with a more or less snake-like appearance.[17]

How had the symptom become entrenched? At this point Breuer underlined its constant conjunction with Anna's absences. Her contracture and other symptoms as well had set in during short absences. Breuer attributed to them—her hypnoid states, to use the technical term he devised—the persistent power of certain emotionally charged ideas. An idea arising in such a state, he claimed, remained "exempt from being worn away by thought"; it remained "withdrawn from 'associative contact'" that would have weakened it, rendering it innocuous. And as Anna's absences increased, so too did the tenacity of her symptoms. It was "only after she had begun to pass more time in her *condition seconde* than in her normal state, that the hysterical phenomena . . . changed from intermittent acute symptoms into chronic ones."[18]

Thus a powerful idea could produce somatic phenomena, just "as the big snake hallucinated by Anna . . . started her contracture"—which figured as a prime example of "conversion."[19] The expression itself, Breuer implied, originated with Freud; the conception, his collaborator insisted, came to them "simultaneously and together."[20] What it signified was, in Freud's words, "the transformation of psychical excitation into . . . somatic symptoms."[21] Breuer speculated at some length about how such a transformation was wrought—without making headway. He did feel certain, however, that conversion took place most readily during hypnoid states. In such states the body was at the mercy of the psyche.

.   .   .

Baroness Fanny Moser, alias Emmy von N., was about forty years of age when she was referred to Freud.[22] In writing up the case, Freud shifted her geographical origin from German-speaking Switzerland to the partly German-speaking Baltic provinces of Russia. Her social position remained unaffected by this shift: in both Freud's account and in actuality her family had possessed large estates, and in her early twenties she had married a rich industrialist considerably older than herself. After a short marriage her husband had died of a heart attack, leaving her with two daughters, one aged about two, the other having just been born. That was fourteen years before she encountered Freud. In the interval illness "with varying degrees of severity"—temporarily relieved "by a course of massage combined with electric baths"—had been her lot. Her most recent bout of depression, sleeplessness, and tormenting pains had brought her to the Austrian capital. Having spent six weeks in Vienna "in the care of a physician of outstanding merit"—most likely Breuer—she began seeing Freud in May 1889.[23]

Freud treated Emmy for approximately seven weeks, starting on May 1; a year later she returned to Vienna, and he treated her for another eight weeks. It was the first period—more precisely the first eighteen days—that he narrated in detail, "reproducing the notes" he "made each evening."[24] Like Breuer in the case of Anna O., Freud devoted an enormous amount of time to Emmy, usually visiting her twice a day for hypnosis and massage. At the end of this first period, Emmy declared that she had not felt so well since her husband's death and left Vienna in an optimistic frame of mind. Seven months later Breuer, not Freud, received distressing news of her elder daughter's nervous troubles and her own relapse. Almost exactly a year after her first meeting with Freud, she was again in Vienna and again in his hands. In general Emmy proved to be less ill than she had been the previous year, and this second period of treatment apparently also produced good but not lasting results. About her subsequent history Freud said little; it seems clear that she remained nervous and eccentric.

Where Breuer had used Anna O.'s autohypnotic states to investigate the origin of her symptoms, Freud relied on hypnosis itself. Emmy was, he wrote, "an excellent subject for hypnotism." He "had only to hold up a finger in front of her and order her to go to sleep, and she sank back with a dazed . . . look." Gradually her features relaxed and "took on a peaceful appearance." When she awoke, "she looked about her for a moment in a confused way . . . and then became quite lively and on the spot"—and could not remember what had gone on while she had been hypnotized. In no sense did Freud consider her abnormal when in that condition. Nor did he consider her supernormal. Under hypnosis, she was "subject to all the mental failings" one associated with normal consciousness.[25]

What did rank as abnormal was delirium. In such a state "there was a limitation of consciousness . . . hallucinations and illusions were facilitated to the highest degree and feeble-minded or even nonsensical inferences were made." At the beginning of the treatment the delirium had lasted all day long; thereafter the condition improved so rapidly that it ceased being noticeable. Freud's observations were in fact fullest during the first session. Every two or three minutes, in the midst of conducting an otherwise perfectly coherent conversation, Emmy's face became contorted "into an expression of horror and disgust," and she would break off, stretch out her hands, "spreading and crooking her fingers," and exclaim, "in a changed voice, charged with anxiety":

> "Keep still!—Don't say anything!—Don't touch me!" . . . These interpolations came to an end with equal suddenness and the patient took up what she had been saying, without pursuing her momentary excitement

any further, and without explaining or apologizing for her behaviour—probably, therefore, without herself having noticed the interpolation.[26]

What bearing did these delirious states have on Emmy's conversion symptoms? Did the latter, as Breuer claimed was the case with Anna O., arise in an altered state of consciousness? Freud focused on two in particular. The first were verbal ejaculations, including those already mentioned. Under hypnosis, when asked what they meant, Emmy narrated the experiences from which "Don't touch me!" derived:

> When her brother had been so ill from taking a lot of morphine—she was nineteen at the time—he used often to seize hold of her; and . . . another time, an acquaintance had suddenly gone mad in the house and had caught her by the arm (there was a third, similar instance, which she did not remember exactly); and lastly, . . . when she was twenty-eight and her daughter was very ill, the child had caught hold of her so forcibly in its delirium that she was almost choked. Though these four instances were so widely separated in time, she told . . . them in a single sentence and in such rapid succession that they might have been a single episode in four acts.[27]

Had Emmy been in an altered state of consciousness? "Keep still!"—"Don't say anything!" was presumably just a variation; it suggested the influence of some frightening, indeed hallucinatory, thoughts as well as a confusional state. Beyond that Freud did not go. When Emmy returned to Vienna and to Freud for a second period of treatment, she presented another verbal ejaculation: "She kept pressing her hands to her forehead and calling out in yearning and helpless tones the name 'Emmy,' which was her elder daughter's as well as her own." Since this new exclamation "had only just come into existence," its analysis seemed especially promising.[28]

It became amply apparent that the incantation, rather than originating during a phase of altered consciousness, represented an attempt to ward off a state of that very sort. At the outset of her second period of treatment, Emmy had complained of "storms in her head," and it was when the storms were raging fiercely that she kept calling out her and her child's name. Under hypnosis she informed Freud that he was witnessing a repetition of a scene frequently enacted during her daughter's recent illness. When, in a despairing state, "she felt her thoughts becoming confused, she made it a practice to call out her daughter's name, so that it might help her back to clear-headedness. . . . However chaotic everything else in her head" might be, she wanted to keep her thoughts about her daughter "free from confusion."[29] Her protective formula had obviously failed to accomplish its purpose.

The second conversion symptom that intrigued Freud, though part of Emmy's regular speech, was itself nonverbal. The symptom, a clacking sound, which Freud claimed defied imitation, was also difficult to describe; it consisted of a "succession of sounds which were convulsively emitted and separated by pauses."[30] Freud had noticed it during his first interview with Emmy—it could not have failed to catch his attention, so frequent and so obtrusive was the noise. He noticed it again when she began treatment with him a second time.

Under what circumstances had the symptom made its first appearance? Once more Freud resorted to hypnosis to question his patient. Emmy replied that she had had the tic-like clacking sound for "the last five years, ever since a time when she was sitting by the bedside of her younger daughter who was very ill, and had wanted to keep absolutely *quiet.*" Instead, as if against her will, she had made the noise. Freud "tried to reduce the importance of the memory" by pointing out to Emmy that "after all nothing had happened to her daughter."[31] This exercise in hypnotic suggestion only partially relieved the symptom.

How had it become ingrained? Freud surmised that it "had come to be attached not solely to the initial" trauma, but to a "long chain of memories associated" with that trauma—memories which he failed to wipe out. "Having originated at a moment of violent fright," it was "thenceforward joined to *any* fright."[32] Neither its initial appearance nor its chronicity seemed to have been contingent upon an altered state of consciousness.

When Freud came to discuss this particular conversion symptom, he introduced the notion of a conflict between the patient's intention and an antithetic idea. In a short paper with a long title, "A Case of Successful Treatment by Hypnotism with Some Remarks on the Origin of Hysterical Symptoms Through Counter-Will" (1892–93), Freud explained at some length what consequences antithetic ideas, that is, ideas contrary to a person's conscious intention, might produce. Someone enjoying "the powerful self-confidence of health" would suppress and inhibit them, excluding "them from his associations"— often with such success that no sign of their existence would become manifest. In contrast, someone suffering from a nervous state, very generally conceived of as a "tendency to depression and to a lowering of self-confidence," would pay great attention to such ideas—thereby intensifying them. It was when an antithetic idea, now pathologically intensified, became disconnected from consciousness—as happened in hysteria—that it could "put itself into effect by innervation of the body just as easily as . . . a volitional idea in normal circumstances." "The antithetic idea establishes itself, so to speak, as a *'counter-will';* while the patient is aware with astonishment of having a will which is resolute but powerless."[33]

Freud seemed intent on distancing himself from Breuer's notion of hypnoid states. He found, however, no clear substitute; he made no systematic attempt to explore how antithetic ideas became disconnected from consciousness. In Emmy's case history, he borrowed the "terminology of Janet and his followers" to invoke a partially exhausted "primary" ego.[34] As for conversion itself, that is, for the transformation of psychical excitation into somatic symptoms, its status remained unquestioned.

.　　　.　　　.

In contrast to Anna O., Ilona Weiss, alias Elisabeth von R., did not suffer from absences; unlike Emmy von N., she did not suffer from delirium.[35] She was not even a good subject for hypnotism. Early in the treatment, Freud proposed to put her "into a deep hypnosis" and failed. He expressed gratitude that his patient had not gloated over his failure. (On occasion, however, his efforts met with success. At points where "some link . . . would be missing," he would "penetrate into deeper layers of her memories . . . by carrying out an investigation under hypnosis or by the use of some similar technique": applying pressure to Elisabeth's head was what he had in mind).[36] Altered states of consciousness, then, were central neither to her illness nor to Freud's treatment of it—a treatment whose outcome he regarded as a cure.

What were her hysterical symptoms? When in the autumn of 1892 Freud first examined Elisabeth, she complained of pains in her legs which "had developed gradually during the previous two years," which "varied greatly in intensity," and which made walking and even standing difficult.

A fairly large, ill-defined area of the anterior surface of the right thigh was indicated as the focus of the pains. . . . In this area the skin and muscles were also particularly sensitive to pressure and pinching (though the prick of a needle was . . . met with a certain amount of unconcern). This hyperalgesia of the skin and muscles was not restricted to this area but could be observed more or less over the whole of both legs. The muscles were perhaps even more sensitive . . . than the skin; but there could be no question that the thighs were the parts most sensitive to both these kinds of pain.[37]

Freud did not find it easy to arrive at a differential diagnosis. What persuaded him to regard Elisabeth as a case of hysteria—aside from having had no reason to think she was suffering from "any serious organic affection"—was her description of the pains. Their indefiniteness stood in marked contrast to the specificity supplied by someone with an organic ailment. With such patients, Freud continued, if one stimulated the painful area, their faces took on "an expression of discomfort." With Elisabeth the expression "was one of pleasure . . .— her face flushed, she threw back her head and shut her eyes and her body bent backwards."[38] This response could be reconciled only with the view that the stimulation had touched the bodily zone centrally implicated in what Freud now labeled hysteria.

Having made a diagnosis, he approached Elisabeth's case with quite definite hopes and expectations. He aimed, he wrote, "to grasp the connection between the events of her illness and her actual symptom." By "events of her illness" he meant emotionally charged scenes, and the emotional component itself had a distinct shape in his mind. With Emmy's case before him, he awaited an account by his new patient of a conflict-ridden experience and the consequent unmasking of an antithetic or incompatible idea. He had heard a great deal of her narrative and reported it—so fully that he found his case history "read" like a short story—before he was satisfied that he had understood those "events."[39]

To Freud, Elisabeth's tale initially seemed composed of "commonplace emotional upheavals." The youngest of three daughters, she had been her father's favorite, or at least the one her father claimed "took the place of a son and friend with whom he could exchange ideas." She herself was "greatly discontented with being a girl": she wanted to study; she wanted to have musical training; "she was indignant at the idea of having to sacrifice her inclinations and her freedom of judgement by marriage." When the daughters became nubile, the family moved from its Hungarian estates to Vienna. Not long thereafter it endured a series of devastating blows. First, Elisabeth's father died, after an eighteen-month illness during which "she played the leading part at his sick-bed."[40] Next, she repeated that role in nursing her mother through several bouts of ill-health, which the older woman survived. By then her two sisters were married, the elder to someone not to Elisabeth's liking, the second to someone congenial. The final blow struck when the second sister died in childbirth before Elisabeth and her mother could arrive to bid her farewell.

Freud was far from satisfied: no scene or scenes of emotional conflict stood out in this bare recital. He determined to persevere, and to make Elisabeth persevere. He applied pressure to her head and instructed her to tell him what came to mind at that very moment. "She remained silent for a long time and then, on my insistence, admitted that she had thought of an evening on which a young man had seen her home after a party, of the conversation that had taken place between them and of the feelings with which she had returned home to her father's sick-bed." The young man, it emerged, had long been "devotedly attached to her father and . . . had extended his admiration to the ladies of the family"—particularly to Elisabeth. And she had responded. Here was someone, she secretly thought, with whom the idea of marriage was a source of pleasure rather than of indignation. No formal understanding, however, existed between them. Her romantic hopes reached a climax on the night she now recalled—and then, returning home in a "blissful frame of mind," she had found her father much worse. (Thereafter she never left him for an entire evening and seldom saw the young man.) Here Freud discerned the requisite "situation of incompatibility": Elisabeth's blissful feeling on the one hand; her father's deteriorating condition, and the self-reproaches it prompted, on the other.[41]

This was not the only such scene Freud unearthed. A second scene of equal or even greater conflict emerged toward the end of the treatment. By the time Elisabeth recounted it, Freud had already detected his patient's affection for her second sister's husband. Elisabeth herself remained in the dark; she "continued to reproduce her recollections" unaware of what they were revealing. She recalled the alarming news about her sister and the long journey with her mother to the summer resort where her sister lived,

> reaching there in the evening, the hurried walk through the garden to the door of the small . . . house, the silence within and the oppressive darkness; how her brother-in-law was not there to receive them, and how they stood before the bed and looked at her sister as she lay there dead. At that moment of dreadful certainty that her beloved sister was dead . . .—at that very moment another thought had shot through Elisabeth's mind, and now forced itself irresistibly upon her once more, like a flash of lightning in the dark: "Now he is free again and I can be his wife."[42]

By this time Freud was convinced that he had located the events of Elisabeth's illness, understood as antithetic or incompatible ideas. How did they link to her actual symptoms? What figured as crucial in Freud's mind—and here he was in agreement with Breuer—was the fact that "an ideational group with so much emotional emphasis" had been kept isolated, that is, "cut off from any free associative connection . . . with the rest of the . . . content of her mind." But he resorted to neither Breuer's hypnoid states nor the "terminology of Janet and his followers" in accounting for this isolation. Instead he introduced a notion that was to rank as constitutive of the psychoanalytic domain— the notion of defense. It was the patient's act of will in fending off the incompatible idea that led to "the formation of a separate psychical group." It was "the refusal on the part of the patient's ego to come to terms" with such an idea that rendered the idea a "body . . . foreign" to consciousness yet acting upon it.[43]

The introduction of defense represented only a first step. Freud took a second step when he called on conversion. The first step marked a divergence from Breuer; the second (since the concept was shared) provoked no difficulties with his colleague. The difficulties Freud encountered came in trying to fit conversion with the history of this particular patient. Again using Emmy's case as exemplar, Freud had set out to identify the scene at which "the conversion occurred."[44] He had identified more than one emotionally charged scene, but he had found no conversion. In the first scene, the pains failed to make an appearance; by the time of the second, they had already become manifest.

Freud backtracked. He set out again, this time in pursuit of Elisabeth's pains. During the time she was nursing her father, she had frequently "jumped out of bed with bare feet in a cold room," and, in fact, "in addition to complaining about the pain in her legs she also complained of tormenting sensations of cold." During that period, however, she could remember only "a single attack of pain, which had lasted . . . a day or two." It was two years later, while on holiday with her extended family, now reconstituted after her father's death and her sisters' marriages, that her "pains and locomotor weakness started" in earnest. From this chronology Freud was led to conclude that what began as a "mild rheumatic affection" subsequently provided the "model copied" in Elisabeth's hysteria.[45]

The events and the pains had not coincided in the past as Freud had anticipated. They coincided in the present in a way he had not foreseen. Elisabeth's painful legs, he wrote, "began to 'join in the conversation.'"

> As a rule the patient was free from pain when we started work. If, then, by a question or by pressure upon her head I called up a memory, a sensation of pain would make its first appearance, and this was usually so sharp that the patient would give a start and put her hand to the painful spot. The pain that was thus aroused would persist so long as she was under the influence of the memory; it would reach its climax when she was in the act of telling me the essential and decisive part of what she had to communicate, and with the last word . . . it would disappear.

In this way, Freud asserted, he obtained "a plastic impression" of the fact that the somatic symptom took the place of a psychical excitation, "exactly as the conversion theory of hysteria" claimed.[46]

His enthusiasm for conversion theory did not last. Though he never publicly distanced himself from it, he let it languish. By 1909 he had come to regard hysterical conversion as a "leap from a mental process to a somatic innervation" that could "never be fully comprehensible."[47] By 1926 he had come to the conclusion that this incomprehensibility offered "a good reason for quitting such an unproductive field without delay."[48]

In itself the notion of conversion had not proved unproductive. It had invited the body to enter a domain that was in the process of being defined as unconscious. The invitation had been indirect, the kind of invitation one extends to the significant other of an intended guest. What would happen if Freud tried a direct approach—that is, if he started from the soma rather than from the psyche?

Soma and Psyche

In his paper entitled "Sexuality in the Aetiology of the Neuroses" (1898), Freud narrated a case that had displayed "a puzzling alternation" of symptoms. The young man in question had been sent by his physician to a hydropathic establishment "on account of a typical neurasthenia" with symptoms of "intercranial pressure, fatigue, and dyspepsia." Initially his condition showed a steady and marked improvement, "so that there was every prospect . . . he would be discharged as a grateful disciple of hydrotherapy. But in the sixth week a complete change occurred; the patient 'could no longer tolerate the water'"; he became "more and more nervous"—suffering from "attacks of dyspnoea, vertigo in walking, and disturbances of sleep." After two more weeks the afflicted young man left the establishment, "uncured and dissatisfied."

An accurate description of the symptoms was all Freud needed to solve the mystery. With an air of triumph he lectured the young man, who was now his patient, on his sexual history.

> "As you yourself very well know, you fell ill as a result of long-continued masturbation. In the sanatorium you gave up this form of satisfaction, and therefore you quickly recovered. When you felt well, however, you unwisely sought to have relations with a lady—a fellow-patient, let us suppose—which could only lead to excitement without normal satisfaction. . . . It was this relationship, not a sudden inability to tolerate hydrotherapy, which caused you to fall ill once more. Moreover, your present state of health leads me to conclude that you are continuing this relationship here in town as well." I can assure my readers that the patient confirmed what I had said, point by point.[49]

In both phases the young man was suffering from what Freud called an actual neurosis—that is, the etiology was of a "present-day kind," in contrast to hysteria, where the prime etiological factor was located in the past. (The two such neuroses that Freud diagnosed in this case were neurasthenia and anxiety neurosis.) In both phases that factor

36

could have been discovered simply by questioning the patient. It could have been discovered even without questioning the patient. After all, Freud had proceeded directly from the symptoms to their cause. "The morphology," he wrote, could "with little difficulty be translated into aetiology."[50] The challenge lay not in linking symptoms and sexual practices, but in sexuality itself.

In turning to sexuality to account for the etiology of the neuroses in general and of the actual neuroses in particular, Freud forthwith conscripted the body into the unconscious domain. Breuer once again disagreed. He regarded his younger colleague's single-minded insistence with dismay and as likely to do him "a lot of harm."[51] At least this was the attitude Freud attributed to Breuer and reported to Wilhelm Fliess. In turning to sexuality, Freud was also turning to Fliess.

When their "congress" in Achensee—held in the summer of 1900 and the last of such meetings, once eagerly anticipated as occasions for a free and frank exchange of ideas—had ended in acrimony, Freud wrote Fliess lamenting the loss of his "audience." For whom, he dolefully inquired, would he now write?[52] For whom had he been writing during the previous decade? (Strong claims have been advanced for Fliess's influence on Freud, claims that documentary lacunae make difficult to assess.[53] The so-called Freud-Fliess correspondence, which provides abundant evidence of Freud's conceptual vicissitudes in the 1890s, is only half a correspondence; the Fliess letters are lacking, and hence it is impossible to locate precisely his contribution to those vicissitudes.) The two had met in the autumn of 1887, when Fliess, on a visit to Vienna for professional study, heeded Breuer's advice and attended Freud's lectures on neurology. Fliess's own expertise lay in the nose and throat, and until the end of his life he enjoyed a flourishing practice in Berlin. But his otolaryngological knowledge constituted merely a point of departure for interests that extended over a far wider area. From the testimony of his acquaintances and from his own writings, Fliess emerges as a "remarkable, indeed fascinating" personality (Freud's words),[54] endowed with a "fondess for far-reaching speculation," and possessed of "a wealth of biological knowledge."[55] It was this last that Freud hoped to exploit.

These hopes reached their most feverish pitch when Fliess was developing his periodicity theory.[56] In *Beyond the Pleasure Principle*

(1920) Freud retrospectively summarized and then dismissed the sweeping "conception of Wilhelm Fliess" according to which "all phenomena of life exhibited by organisms—and no doubt, their death—" were "linked with the completion of fixed periods" themselves dependent upon two kinds of living substance, one female, one male.[57] Apart from the menstrual cycle of twenty-eight days, Fliess had argued that another "group of periodic phenomena" existed "with a twenty-three day cycle." People of all ages and both sexes were subject to these two.

> A mother transmits her periods to her child and determines its sex by the period which is first transmitted. The periods then continue in the child, and are repeated with the same rhythm from generation to generation. They can no more be created anew than can energy, and their rhythm survives as long as organised beings reproduce themselves sexually.[58]

In the mid-1890s Freud had been intrigued, rather than put off, by the "rigidity of Fliess's formulas."[59] He expressed excitement at the prospect of "dealing with something" that would "cement" his and his friend's work, that would place his own "structure" on Fliess's "base." He expressed excitement at the prospect that with his friend's help he would discover "solid ground"; he would "cease to give psychological explanations and begin to find a physiological foundation!" Elsewhere he voiced a fervent wish to build jointly with Fliess, blending their contributions to the point where their "individual property" would no longer be "recognizable." Before long, however, his tone changed: he confessed to his friend that he was baffled.

> I am not at all in disagreement with you, not at all inclined to leave the psychology hanging in the air without an organic base. But apart from this conviction I do not know how to go on. . . . Why I cannot fit it together [the organic and the psychological] I have not even begun to fathom.[60]

Though Freud's dream of collaboration with Fliess remained unfulfilled, his association with the Berlin otolarygologist left an indelible imprint on him. It was Fliess who reinforced Freud's turn toward infantile sexuality if he did not actually point the way; after all, his periodicity theory implied its existence.[61] Yet it was Freud, not Fliess, who appreciated that sexuality made a "demand upon . . . the mind for work."[62]

.   .   .

Frau Emmy von N. "exhibited only a small amount of conversion." Her verbal ejaculations and her clacking sound fitted under that rubric, but were themselves only a minor part of her rich symptomatology. The far more numerous psychical—as opposed to somatic—symptoms Freud "divided into alterations of mood . . . phobias and abulias (inhibitions of will)."[63] In his paper "On the Grounds for Detaching a Particular Syndrome from Neurasthenia Under the Description 'Anxiety Neurosis'" (1895), Emmy's psychical symptoms, more particularly her phobias, led to her selection, without her name being mentioned, as a clinical example of "anxious expectation."[64]

In *Studies on Hysteria* Freud laid stress on the traumatic origins of Emmy's phobias. Her fear of animals of all sizes and shapes loomed large, and Freud repeatedly induced her to tell what he called "animal stories," that is, to narrate the frightening experiences she had undergone in which animals had figured. And then he "tried to free her" from her fears by going over each animal and asking her if she was still afraid of it. Sometimes she answered "no"; sometimes she replied that she "mustn't be afraid"—a procedure Freud came to regard as altogether inadequate and superficial.[65] In his paper on anxiety neurosis, he was less interested in the origins of a particular phobia than in the patient's susceptibility to trauma. In both texts he suggested that to account for such susceptibility, the notion of "anxious expectation" or "a tendency to anxiety" should be introduced. He further claimed that this expectation or tendency derived from "the fact that the patient had been living for years in a state of sexual abstinence."[66]

To detach anxiety neurosis from neurasthenia, Freud needed to establish an etiology and to distinguish it from that of neurasthenia. He had already postulated masturbation as the sexual etiology for neurasthenia; hence he needed to establish a different sexual etiology for anxiety neurosis. To that end he "brought together the cases" in which he had "found anxiety arising from a sexual cause," and as he made a survey of his patients and segregated them in categories, he implicitly reckoned Emmy among the intentionally abstinent.[67]

The cases appeared "quite heterogeneous."[68] At the same time they epitomized the sociology of late nineteenth-century, mostly bourgeois, mostly "normal," sexual practice. In Draft E, entitled "How Anxiety Originates," which Freud sent Fliess in 1894, as well as in the paper published the following year, he analyzed his sample first by sex and then by age. The youngest group of women had succumbed to *"virginal anxiety"*—virginal men also ran a risk, but a smaller one. "A number of unambiguous observations" had convinced Freud that anxiety neurosis could be produced in adolescent girls "by their first encounter with the problem of sex, by any more or less sudden revelation of what had till then been hidden—for instance, by witnessing the sexual act, or being told or reading about these things." Marriage offered no respite. On the contrary: Freud devised a category of *"anxiety in the newly-married"* for women who "remained anaesthetic during their first cohabitations." Fortunately for them, as soon as the anaesthesia "gave place to normal sensitivity," the anxiety neurosis disappeared. Not so fortunate were those married women whose husbands suffered from "ejaculatio praecox or from markedly impaired potency," or whose husbands practiced "coitus interruptus or reservatus." What linked these impairments and practices was the likelihood that the women involved would be deprived of "satisfaction in coitus. . . . Coitus reservatus by *means of condoms*," for example, would not be "injurious to the woman, provided" she was "very quickly excitable and the husband very potent."[69] Then came anxiety in widows and other "*intentionally abstinent* people" (this category included men as well as women), particularly those who regarded "everything sexual as horrible"—and here Freud probably had Emmy in mind.[70] Finally there were those suffering from "anxiety in the *climacteric*": anxiety due to "the last major increase of sexual need."[71]

In sorting through his male sample, Freud enumerated only three age-related categories. The first comprised those whose anxiety derived from "a state of *unconsummated excitation*," a state Freud associated with "the period of engagement before marriage"—his own engagement had lasted four years. Here he found "the purest cases of the neurosis." Marriage itself entailed risks, though less so for men than for women. Again coitus interruptus figured prominently, and again the nub of the matter was satisfaction in coitus. Coitus interruptus, Freud claimed, was injurious to the man only if, in order to give his partner pleasure, he directed "coitus voluntarily" and postponed "emission."[72] Still more threatened was the man who did not "employ" his "erection for coitus" at all. Here Freud expressed doubts about the purity of the resulting anxiety neurosis: it was likely to be mixed with neurasthenia. Finally there was anxiety linked to old age: the anxiety of men who went *"beyond their desire or strength."*[73] Under this rubric Freud probably included "a jolly old bachelor" he had seen, who produced "a classic anxiety attack after he let himself be seduced by his thirty-year-old mistress into having intercourse three times in a row."[74]

Was there a common element, Freud asked, in this collection? The case of Mr. K., a twenty-four-year-old suffering from anxiety neurosis, about which Freud reported to Fliess in Draft F, suggested an answer. Nine months prior to consulting Freud, he had begun to sleep badly, frequently waking "with night terrors and palpitations." At roughly the same time he fell prey to "gradually increasing general excitability," which, however, abated during "army maneuvers." Three weeks before the consultation, he had experienced "a sudden attack of anxiety for no apparent reason, with a feeling of congestion from his chest up to his head." Subsequently he had been assailed by similar attacks at his midday meal. "In addition during the last two weeks" he complained of short episodes "of deep depression, resembling complete apathy, lasting barely a few minutes." Finally, he reported "attacks of pressure at the back of the head."

Freud had had no time to question Mr. K. about his sexual history before his patient volunteered the requisite information:

> A year ago he fell in love with a girl who was a flirt; huge shock when he heard she was engaged to someone else. No longer in love now.—Attaches little importance to it.—He went on: he masturbated between 13 and 16 or 17 (seduced at school) to a moderate extent, he claimed. Moderate in sexual intercourse; has used a condom for the last two and a half years for fear of infection; often feels tired after it. He described this kind of intercourse as enforced . . . was very much excited sexually in his relations with the girl (without touching her, or the like). His first attack at night . . . [nine months earlier] was two days after coitus; his first anxiety attack was after coitus on the same evening; since then (three weeks) abstinent—a quiet, mild-mannered, and in other ways healthy man.[75]

What Freud emphasized—putting to one side the family history of nervous disorders—was the *"enfeebled* condition" of Mr. K.'s libido.

It "had been diminishing" for about a year; "the preparations for using a condom" were "enough to make him feel the whole act" was "something forced on him and his enjoyment of it something he was talked into." After coitus he sometimes noticed that he felt "weak"; and then, two days later or, as the case might be, "on the next evening," he had an "attack of anxiety." In short, "*reduced* libido," understood as *"psychic"* insufficiency, figured as crucial.[76]

"The concurrence of *reduced* libido and anxiety neurosis," Freud wrote Fliess, jibed with his theoretical expectations.[77] Mr.K.'s enfeebled libido, Freud hypothesized, prevented the discharge of somatic sexual excitation. In turn lack of discharge led to accumulation. And, finally, anxiety itself arose "by *transformation* out of the accumulated sexual tension."[78]

The linkage between psychical desire and the failure to discharge something physical (let alone the transformation of that something into anxiety) was not self-evident. That linkage hinged on Freud's view of sexuality as psychosexuality:

> In the sexually mature male organism somatic sexual excitation is produced—probably continuously—and periodically becomes a stimulus to the psyche. . . . This somatic excitation is manifested as a pressure on the walls of the seminal vesicles, which are lined with nerve endings; thus this visceral excitation will develop continuously, but it will have to reach a certain height before it is able to overcome the resistance of the intervening path of conduction to the cerebral cortex and express itself as a psychical stimulus. When this has happened, however, the group of sexual ideas which is present in the psyche becomes supplied with energy and there comes into being the psychical state of libidinal tension which brings with it an urge to remove that tension. A psychical unloading of this kind is only possible by means of what I shall call *specific* or *adequate* action.[79]

Could a model featuring "pressure on the walls of the seminal vesicles" account for the sexual process in women? Freud claimed that "in essentials" this formula covered both sexes, "in spite," he added, "of the confusion introduced into the problem by all the artificial retarding and stunting of the female sexual instinct." "In women too we must postulate a somatic sexual excitation and a state in which this excitation becomes a psychical stimulus—libido—and provokes the urge to the specific action to which voluptuous feeling is attached." Freud was prepared to acknowledge, however, that where women were concerned, he was "not in a position to say what the process analogous to the relaxation of tension of the seminal vesicles" might be.[80]

Theory and case histories now dovetailed. With "*psychic* enfeeblement" as the quarry, Freud reviewed Mr. K.'s sexual past to answer the question of how that enfeeblement had been acquired.

> There is not much to be got from masturbation in his youth; it would certainly not have had such a result, nor does it seem to have exceeded the usual amount. His relations with the girl, who excited him very much sensually, seem far better suited to produce a disturbance in the required direction; in fact, the case approaches the conditions in the familiar neuroses of men during [long] engagements. But above all, it cannot be disputed that fear of infection and the decision to use a condom laid the foundation. . . . In short, Mr. K. has incurred psychic sexual weakness because he spoiled coitus for himself, and his physical health and production of sexual stimuli being unimpaired, the situation gave rise to the generation of anxiety.[81]

The case of the jolly old bachelor could be explicated in a similar fashion. To most observers, and probably to the patient himself, it might have seemed that his anxiety could be explained by physical exhaustion—with no question being raised about the extent of his psychical stimulation. Freud took an opposite tack. He implied that the jolly old bachelor's anxiety derived from the fact that his somatic arousal had been greater than his psychical, that he had been somatically stirred up without being psychically in the mood. Though he had ejaculated, indeed more than once, a psychic insufficiency had so reduced the quality of his orgasms that somatic sexual excitation was incompletely discharged. As with Mr. K., the result was an inadequate unburdening of that excitation.[82]

In the cases of women also, theory and story dovetailed—despite their lack of seminal vesicles. Take "Katharina," an innkeeper's daughter whom Freud had encountered on a mountain-climbing excursion in the summer of 1893, who figured in *Studies on Hysteria* and stood as an example of virginal anxiety.[83] (Her hysterical symptom, he claimed, "repeated" one created by an initial anxiety neurosis.)[84] At the age of fourteen, that is, four years before meeting Freud, an uncle (years later Freud disclosed that he had disguised the girl's father in this fashion) had attempted on several occasions to force himself upon her sexually, and two years later, at the age of sixteen, she had seen the same uncle lying on top of a cousin. At this point the notion of sexual intercourse had entered Katharina's head, and simultaneously her symptom—a shortness of breath, so sharp that at times she thought she would suffocate—appeared. The notion had entered her head accompanied by the memory of how she had "felt her uncle's body" when he had pressed himself against her.[85] Once again, Freud suggested, a discrepancy and a failure of linkage between the somatic and the psychical accounted for the anxiety attack: at sixteen the memory aroused Katharina somatically (at fourteen she was still "pre-sexual," and hence the experience itself had failed to stir her),[86] but the "group of ideas to which the somatic sexual excitation" should have "become attached" was "not yet enough developed."[87]

Emmy scarcely had a sexual story at all; hers was a tale of abstinence. Abstinence, in Freud's view, amounted to the "withholding of the specific action" which ordinarily followed "upon libido."[88] Such withholding might well produce both an accumulation of somatic excitation and a decline in libido—one either used libido or lost it. Anxiety neurosis constituted only part of Emmy's clinical picture, and not the part that Freud emphasized. Her case raised, as did Katharina's, the question of the similarities between anxiety neurosis, now detached from neurasthenia, and conversion hysteria.

When Freud compared the two, the resemblances turned out to be striking:

> In the latter [hysteria] just as in the former [anxiety neurosis] we find a *psychical insufficiency, as a consequence of which abnormal somatic processes arise*. In the latter just as in the former, too, instead of a psychical working-over of the excitation, a deflection of it occurs into the somatic field; the difference is merely that in anxiety neurosis the excitation . . . is purely somatic . . . whereas in hysteria it is psychical.[89]

One might also add that the rules of conversion and of transformation alike were to prove intractable.[90]

Still Freud persevered. He never gave up on the body. Instead, with the notion of sexuality as psychosexual at his disposal, he reconceptualized the body itself.

.   .   .

When Freud had stimulated the painful area of Elisabeth von R.'s legs, she had cried out; but noticing her closed eyes, "her body bent backwards," and a pleasurable expression on her face, he "could not help thinking that . . . she was having a voluptuous tickling sensation."[91] He had touched a zone which, following the French neuropathologist Jean-Martin Charcot, he designated as hysterogenic. (Elsewhere he defined such zones as "supersensitive areas of the body, on which a slight stimulus" released "an [hysterical] attack.")[92] How, he wondered, could this zone have come into being?

Freud felt satisfied that as far as Elisabeth's right leg was concerned, he had solved the puzzle—or rather that his patient had solved it for him. She had informed him, after recalling the first scene of emotional conflict, that "she now knew why it was that the pains always radiated from the particular area of the right thigh and were at their most painful there: it was in this place that her father used to rest his leg every morning, while she renewed the bandage round it, for it was badly swollen." It was this "associative connection" that Freud regarded as crucial: it had exerted "a positively decisive influence" on the emergence of "an atypical hysterogenic zone."[93] By the same token that zone had been established by chance.

What transformed the accidental and barely sexual hysterogenic into the foreordained and sexually saturated erotogenic was Freud's dawning appreciation that psychosexuality had its origin in infancy. In a letter to Fliess dated December 6, 1896, he had first mentioned the idea that during childhood sexual excitation was produced by "a great many parts of the body," that is, by a variety of erotogenic zones. The following November he returned to the subject at greater length, emphasizing again how, in infancy, sexuality was not yet localized; in small children erotogenic zones which were later abandoned—he pointed specifically to "the regions of the anus and of the mouth and throat"—made a "contribution" to it, in a way that was "analogous" to the "sexual organs proper."[94] An erotogenic zone, then, unlike its hysterogenic cousin, was explicitly bound up with something somatic—indeed, as the mouth and anus would suggest, with a vital bodily function.

Given a somatic basis, how did an erotogenic zone establish itself? The prime exhibit in the *Three Essays on the Theory of Sexuality* was the child's lips. The somatic basis, the need for nourishment, was readily apparent. So too was the pleasurable sensation produced by the "warm flow of milk" which accompanied the satisfaction of that need. "No one," wrote Freud, waxing rhapsodic, "who has seen a baby sinking back satiated from the breast and falling asleep with flushed cheeks and a blissful smile" could "escape the reflection that this picture" persisted "as a prototype of the expression of sexual satisfaction." The next step ranked as crucial: separation of the "need for repeating the sexual satisfaction" from the "need for taking nourishment." As an example Freud cited a child's sucking on "part of his own skin" instead of on an "extraneous body" and the establishment of the labial region as an erotogenic zone that went along with it.[95] In this fashion an erotogenic zone became an archive of experiences of satisfaction; in this fashion an erotogenic zone ceased being determined solely by physiology.

It was not every child, Freud added, who sucked the way he had described, but many of his women patients who suffered from, among other symptoms, "constriction of the throat" had "indulged energetically in sucking during their childhood."[96] Such had been true of "Dora."

In 1894, four years before Freud met Ida Bauer, alias "Dora," and six years before he began treating her, Philip Bauer, her father and a wealthy textile manufacturer, had been in his care. The therapy prescribed had been neither psychological nor psychoanalytic; it had been a vigorous "anti-luetic treatment." Bauer's "confusional attack, followed by symptoms of paralysis and slight mental disturbance," Freud attributed to a syphilitic infection his patient had contracted before his marriage. In fact the father's health had been and remained the family's dominant concern and dictated its place of residence. Freud never met Dora's mother, but gathered from reports of father and daughter alike that she too was afflicted—in her case with "housewife's psychosis." "She had no understanding of her children's more active interests, and was occupied all day long in cleaning the house with its furniture and utensils and in keeping them clean—to such an extent as to make it almost impossible to use or enjoy them." (Dora had one sibling, an older brother, Otto, who became a leader of the Austrian Socialist party.) In 1898 the father "brought his daughter, who had meanwhile grown unmistakably neurotic," for a consultation, and two years later "handed her over" to Freud "for psychoanalytic treatment."[97]

Freud was not the only man to whom Dora's father consigned her. According to Dora—and Freud thought her guilty of only slight exaggeration—"she had been handed over to Herr K. as the price of his tolerating the relations between her father and his [Herr K.'s] wife." Years earlier, that is, shortly after her father's vigorous anti-luetic treatment, it had become clear to the "sharp-sighted Dora" that the friendship between her parents and the Ks merely served as a screen for an affair between her father and Frau K. From the beginning of it Herr K. had sought solace from the daughter of the adulterer. Dora found herself the recipient of flowers and presents, and "in the constant and unsupervised companionship of a man who had no satisfaction from his own wife." To none of this did she object. But she did object, on two occasions, to Herr K.'s importunities. On the first—she was then fourteen—he took advantage of a secluded meeting and "suddenly clasped" her "to him and pressed a kiss upon her lips." Two years later, Dora reported, he "had the audacity to make her a proposal while they were on a walk after a trip" upon a lake.[98] Here, Freud commented, was plentiful material for psychical trauma.

When in October 1900 Dora, now aged eighteen, had begun treatment with Freud, he had written enthusiastically to Fliess about setting to work with his new patient, whose case had "smoothly opened to the existing collection of picklocks."[99] In that collection figured psychical trauma and emotional conflict—hence his initial focus on the two scenes just mentioned. (Here were the "psychological determinants" he had postulated in *Studies on Hysteria*.) He soon discovered that the case would not smoothly open. Less than three months after beginning treatment and before "some of the problems had . . . even been attacked and others had only been imperfectly elucidated," Dora abruptly broke it off. With dreams as a second—and principal focus—Freud set to work again, this time writing up the incomplete analysis. It was, he wrote Fliess, "a fragment of an analysis of a case of hysteria in which the explanations" were "grouped around two dreams." The very brevity of the treatment ranked in his mind as an advantage; had it lasted, say, for a year, he would "not have known how to deal with the material involved."[100] He finished the manuscript in short order and entitled it "Dream and Hysteria." (He reckoned Dora's story a continuation of his own *Interpretation of Dreams*.) But that was not all. It had a third focus: it also contained "glimpses of the organic [elements], that is, the erotogenic zones."[101] For reasons that remain unclear, the fragment was not published until 1905, the same year as the *Three Essays*.

Freud fastened on Dora's nervous cough and aphonia—both conversion symptoms. The cough had made its first appearance, along with migraine headaches, when she was twelve. The migraines grew less frequent and by the time she was sixteen had vanished altogether. Not so the attacks of *tussis nervosa*. When Dora first appeared in Freud's consulting room, she was "suffering from a cough and from hoarseness," and he "proposed giving her psychological treatment." His "proposal was not adopted, since the attack in question, like the others, passed off spontaneously." When she was sent to Freud for treatment two years later, "she was again coughing in a characteristic manner."[102]

In Elisabeth's case Freud had suggested that an organic disorder, a mild rheumatic ailment, had furnished the model copied by her hysteria. In Dora's case he assumed that the "presence of a real and organically determined irritation of the throat . . . acted like the grain of sand around which an oyster forms its pearl." Elsewhere he eschewed metaphor and simply claimed that the nervous cough "had no doubt been started by a common catarrh." In an effort to shed light on what was admittedly obscure, Freud introduced the notion of somatic compliance.

> As far as I can see, every hysterical symptom involves the participation of *both* [somatic and psychical] sides. It cannot occur without the presence of a certain degree of *somatic compliance* offered by some normal or pathological process in or connected with one of the bodily organs. And it cannot occur more than once—and the capacity for repeating itself is one of the characteristics of a hysterical symptom—unless it has a psychical significance, a *meaning*.

Freud underlined how seldom the somatic compliance was forthcoming; it was far more likely that new meanings would accrue to an existing organic condition than that a new condition would appear.

> These remarks would make it seem that the somatic side of a hysterical symptom is the more stable of the two and the harder to replace, while the psychical side is a variable element for which a substitute can more easily be found.[103]

Having inserted somatic compliance, Freud made no further attempt to find an organic key to the formation of hysterical symptoms.

He turned to the psychical side. Dora, he discovered, had been a thumb-sucker, a habit which "had persisted into her fourth or fifth year"; thereafter, he inferred, her throat "had to a high degree re-tained" its erotogenic significance.[104] Given the throat as erotogenic zone, a physical irritation became endowed with meanings.

What meanings? In the narrative of his treatment Freud offered two fully worked-out interpretations.[105] Dora's attacks of coughing and the accompanying aphonia, he suggested, mimicked the behavior of Frau K. (He explored only cursorily, almost as an afterthought, Dora's homosexual love for her father's mistress.)[106] Whenever her husband was away, Frau K. felt fine; whenever he returned, she suddenly fell ill. She was obviously using ill-health to avoid "conjugal duties," and the presence or absence of her husband had a decisive "influence upon the appearance and disappearance of the symptoms of her illness." So much Freud had surmised—and his patient as well. Might not Dora's health be determined in a fashion similar to Frau K.'s?—or rather, in reverse: she was well when Herr K. was present, ill when he was absent. (Freud had already come to the conclusion that Dora secretly loved Herr K.) Freud asked his patient what the average length of her attacks of aphonia had been:

"From three to six weeks, perhaps." How long had Herr K.'s absences lasted? "Three to six weeks, too," she was obliged to admit. Her illness was therefore a demonstration of her love for K., just as his wife's was a demonstration of her *dislike.* . . . And this really seemed to have been so, at least during the first period of the attacks.

How could Dora's illness serve as such a demonstration? "When the man she loved was away," Freud interpreted, "she gave up speaking; speech had lost its value since she could not speak to him." At the same time, writing, which came more easily to her when her speech was impaired, "gained in importance as being the only means of communication in his absence."[107] Freud did not report Dora's response to his interpretation.

He himself was not satisfied. "The explanation of the symptom" which he had "hitherto obtained was far from fulfilling the require-ments" he was "accustomed to make of such explanations." "At least *one* of the meanings of a symptom," he claimed, was "the repre-sentation of a sexual phantasy."

She had once again been insisting that Frau K. only loved her father because he was *"ein vermögender Mann"* [a man of means]. Certain details of the way in which she expressed herself . . . led me to see that behind this phrase its opposite lay concealed, namely, that her father was *"ein unvermögender Mann"* [a man without means]. This could only be meant in a sexual sense—that her father, as a man, was without means, was impotent. Dora confirmed this interpretation . . . whereupon I pointed out the contradiction she was involved in if on the one hand she continued to insist that her father's relation with Frau K. was a common love-affair, and on the other maintained that her father was impotent. . . . Her answer showed that she had no need to admit the contradiction. She knew very well, she said, that there was more than one way of obtaining sexual gratification. . . . I questioned her further, whether she referred to the use of organs other than the genitals for the purpose of sexual intercourse, and she replied in the affirmative. I could then go on to say that . . . she must be thinking of precisely those parts of the body which in her case were in a state of irritation,—the throat and the oral cavity.

When Dora coughed, Freud concluded, she represented fellatio. Dora "tacitly accepted this interpretation," and shortly thereafter her cough—at least for a time—"vanished."[108]

In conceptualizing erotogenic zones, Freud did not intend to sever the connection between the erotogenic and the physiological. The relationship between them had become problematic, and among his collection of picklocks, he possessed none which would allow him to sort that relationship out. Yet he might find that he had at hand ones which would enable him to explore how the erotogenic endowed with meanings not simply physical conditions but the ego itself, and in this fashion transformed it into a "bodily ego."

"A Bodily Ego"

In his paper "The Disposition to Obsessional Neurosis" (1913), Freud recounted the case of "a woman patient whose neurosis underwent an unusual change." It started out as a "straightforward anxiety hysteria," and it "retained that character for a few years. One day, however, it suddenly changed into an obsessional neurosis of the severest type."[109] The sequence proved to be instructive.

In a fashion that had now become familiar to his readers, Freud proceeded to relate the woman's current sexual history:

Up to the time of her falling ill the patient had been a happy and almost completely satisfied wife. She wanted to have children, . . . and she fell ill when she learned that it was impossible for her to have any by the husband who was the only object of her love. . . . Her husband understood, without any admission or explanation on her part, what his wife's anxiety meant; he felt hurt, without showing it, and in turn reacted neurotically by—for the first time—failing in sexual intercourse with her. Immediately afterwards he started on a journey. His wife believed that he had become permanently impotent, and produced her first obsessional symptoms on the day before his expected return.

The obsessional symptoms the patient displayed, "her compulsion for scrupulous washing and cleanliness and extremely energetic protective measures against severe injuries which she thought other people had reason to fear from her," did not at once disclose their connection to her sexual life. That life had itself undergone an unusual change. "Owing to the impotence of the only man of whom there could be any question for her," Freud wrote, "her genital life had lost its value." In its place anal-erotic and sadistic impulses had come to the fore. It was against these impulses, defined as components of sexuality, that his patient had constructed bulwarks—reaction-formations was Freud's technical term. Here he took another step, not, he assured his readers, just on the basis on this single patient. He now postulated that the anal-erotic and sadistic impulses joined together in an organization of sexual life which preceded the primacy of the genital zones (and with that primacy, the disposition to hysteria).[110]

When two years later, in 1915, Freud published a revised edition of the *Three Essays,* he extended his notion of the pregenital. In a new section entitled "The Phases of Development of the Sexual Organization," he introduced an oral as well as a sadistic-anal stage, claiming that the oral preceded the anal in the life of a small child. Eight years later, in 1923, in "The Infantile Genital Organization," he added a further stage, which he called phallic.[111] With this addition, his sequence of pregenital stages—the famous oral, anal, and phallic—was complete: human sexuality found itself subsumed under erotogenic zones.

What did that subsumption signify? In the first instance stages represented a way of grouping component instincts; they suggested that the diverse activities to which Freud had extended the label sexual were pressed into the service of a dominant impulse. In the second instance Freud was offering a developmental account: sexuality could best be portrayed as a progression from one pregenital stage to another, culminating in the genital. (Subsequently he was to warn against construing the sequence too rigidly; stages overlapped, he argued, and each stage left permanent traces.)[112]

The primacy of erotogenic zones in succession had been foreshadowed in 1897.[113] Herewith Freud found in his collection of picklocks what was needed to decipher the relationship, not of the erotogenic and the physiological, but of the erotogenic and the ego. Above all it was when the penis had its turn that the erotogenic endowed the ego with the meaning which most concerned Freud, that is, its *"maleness."*[114]

.   .   .

Insofar as the hypotheses about infantile sexuality that he advanced in the first edition of the *Three Essays* derived from clinical work, the patients were all adults whose own infantile sexuality had been subject to various forms of amnesia and distortion. Freud had heeded Polonius's advice: by indirection he had found direction out; but at the same time he confessed "to a wish for . . . less roundabout proof. Surely," he continued, "there must be a possibility of observing children" and their "sexual wishes and impulses . . . at first hand."[115] By the time he penned these words, his own offspring were well past the infantile stages; the youngest was on the verge of adolescence. So he turned to his followers, to the men and women who were beginning to gather around him after the turn of the century, to those who came together in 1902 to form the Wednesday Psychological Society, and asked them to collect observations on their children. One of its members, the musicologist Max Graf, soon began supplying Freud with information about his son, alias Little Hans.

Graf and his wife—she herself had fallen "ill with a neurosis . . . during her girlhood" and had been treated by Freud—had agreed to experiment with letting their son "grow and express himself without being intimidated. . . . They would use no more coercion than might be absolutely necessary for maintaining good behaviour." In two respects, however, the parents adhered more closely to prevailing cultural practices than to Freudian precepts in the making. When Hans was three and half—the reporting on this "cheerful, amiable, active-minded young fellow" began when he was three—his mother "found him with his hand on his penis" and threatened to summon the doctor to cut off his "wiwi-maker." At about the same age a sister was born, and to prepare for what Freud called "the great event of Hans's life," his parents trotted out the fable of the stork. Shortly before the boy turned five, the tenor of the reporting changed abruptly. He had started "setting . . . problems" for his parents, and the material his father now sent was "material for a case history."[116]

What was the matter with Hans? One day on his way to the public gardens with his nursemaid for his regular outing, he was overcome with anxiety; he began to cry and asked to return home to the comfort of his mother. When questioned, he could not say what he was afraid of. The next day his mother accompanied him; again the anxiety proved overwhelming, forcing him to take refuge in the house. When questioned once more, "after much internal struggling," he replied: *"I was afraid a horse would bite me."* This was the first content of Hans's disorder, which Freud classified as a phobia; it was not the last.

> He was not only afraid of horses biting him . . . but also of carts, furniture-vans, and of buses (their common quality being . . . that they were all heavily loaded), and of horses that started moving, of horses that looked big and heavy, and of horses that drove quickly. . . . [H]e was afraid of horses *falling down,* and consequently incorporated in his phobia everything that seemed likely to facilitate their falling down.[117]

The proliferation of fearful objects, Freud remarked, was and was not the result of psychoanalytic work—work that in this instance was being done by Hans's father, and with a successful outcome. Analysis did not account for the disorder, but it did account for a patient's becoming fully "aware of the products of the disease." The analyst thus found himself in the curious position "of coming to the help of a disease, and procuring it its due of attention." As a consequence the phobia "plucked up courage" and ventured "to show itself." (One is reminded of Elisabeth's legs joining in the conversation.) And it was in large part as a contribution toward understanding "this very frequent form of disorder" that Freud wrote up the case material provided by Hans's father. That was not all. The material, Freud hoped, would speak directly to the hypotheses he had advanced in the *Three Essays* and simultaneously shed light "upon the mental life of children."[118]

Even before the onset of his phobia, Hans had displayed what Freud regarded as the principal trait of his sexual life: "a quite peculiarly lively interest in his wiwi-maker." The boy's "Weltanschauung" first came to the notice of his attentive father on trips to the zoo. "Standing in front of the lion's cage . . . Hans called out in a joyful and excited voice: 'I can see the lion's wiwi-maker.'" When his father drew a picture of a giraffe, the boy complained that its genital organ was not in evidence. "Draw its wiwi-maker too," he insisted. "Draw it yourself," the father replied. Hans complied with a short line, then extended it until it was almost the length of the animal's leg. When the father and son walked past a horse that was urinating, Hans commented: "The horse has got its wiwi-maker underneath like me." And one time when he was at the railroad station and "saw water being let out of an engine," he re-marked: "Oh look . . . the engine is making wiwi." Not long thereafter he formulated the crucial difference between animate and inanimate objects, therewith recognizing he had made a mistake: "A dog and a horse have wiwi-makers, a table and a chair haven't."[119]

In the course of the analysis, his father provided much in the way of enlightenment. It did not extend to sexual intercourse. (Here Freud thought the "educational experiment" had not been carried far enough. The boy should have been told about "the existence of the vagina and of copulation.")[120] Yet Hans had premonitions; he listened, Freud was certain, to the "sensations of his penis." Witness a fantasy he reported to his father: "I was with you at Schönbrunn [the location of the zoo] where the sheep are; and then we crawled through under the ropes, and then we told the policeman at the end of the garden, and he grabbed hold of us." Later that same day Hans remembered having thought something, something forbidden: "I went with you in the train, and we smashed a window and the policeman took us off with him." Hans's father made no interpretation, but Freud did: the fantasies offered a "certain pictorial representation" for a "vague no-tion . . . of something that he might do with his mother" whereby he might take possession of her.[121]

The fantasies contained, Freud continued, a significant detail: Hans portrayed his father "as sharing" in his actions. "I should like," the boy seemed to be saying, "to be doing something with my mother . . . I do not know what it is, but I do know that you [the father] are doing it too." The boy did not always imagine his father playing such a benign role. In a further fantasy Hans offered a different version of both taking possession of his mother and his father's attitude thereto: *"In the night there was a big giraffe in the room and a crumpled one; and the big one called out because I took the crumpled one away from it. Then it stopped calling out; and then I sat down on top of the crumpled one."* This time the father made an interpretation. "The big giraffe," he wrote Freud, was himself, or rather his "big penis (the long neck), and the crumpled giraffe" was his "wife, or rather her genital organ."

> The whole thing is a reproduction of a scene which has been gone through almost every morning for the last few days. Hans always comes to us in the early morning, and my wife cannot resist taking him into bed with her for a few minutes. Thereupon I always begin to warn her not to take him into bed with her ("the big one called out because I'd taken the crumpled one away from it"); and she answers now and then, rather irritated, no doubt, that it's all nonsense, that after all one minute is of no importance, and so on. Then Hans stays with her a little while. ("Then the big giraffe stopped calling out; and then I sat down on top of the crumpled one.")[122]

Freud concurred. (Two days later, when the father took Hans for the one and only consultation with his mentor, Freud had a chance to elaborate. He told the boy that long before his birth he had known that "a little Hans would come" into the world "who would be so fond of his mother that he would be bound to feel afraid of his father." Freud then "partly interpreted" the boy's fear of horses for him: "the horse must be his father.")[123]

In a conversation with his father, which focused on big animals, their wiwi-makers, and on the correlation of size of animal and size of wiwi-maker, Hans concluded: "And every one has a wiwi-maker. And my wiwi-maker will get bigger as I get bigger; it's fixed in, of course." The boy now, so Freud's gloss ran, was "oppressed by the fear of having to lose this precious piece of his ego." When his mother had threatened to call the doctor to cut it off, the threat had had no effect. Its effect was "deferred" until a year and a quarter later. Even in the absence of an actual threat, Hans's fear would have been aroused thanks to a bit of sexual enlightenment which only recently had been given him. His father had told him that women did not have penises. (Since he did not specify what they did have, the boy was left to imagine the adult female genital as a crumpled giraffe.) Hans himself had observed his baby sister in the bath and had assumed that her diminutive wiwi-maker would grow in time. The idea that it was not a wiwi-maker at all, he at first found unacceptable. "Could it be," Freud wrote, trying to verbalize the boy's musings, "that living beings really did exist which did not possess wiwi-makers? If so, it would no longer be . . . incredible that they could take his own wiwi-maker away, and, as it were, make him into a woman!"[124]

The doctor might come; he might take away Hans's penis "—but only to give him a bigger one in exchange for it." Such was the fantasy the boy reported at the very end of the treatment.

> *"The plumber came; and first he took away my behind with a pair of pincers, and then gave me another, and then the same with my wiwi-maker.* He said: 'Let me see your behind!' and I had to turn round, and he took it away, and then he said: 'Let me see your wiwi-maker!'"
> Hans's father grasped the nature of the wishful phantasy, and did not hesitate a moment as to the only interpretation it could bear.
> *I:* "He gave you a *bigger* wiwi-maker and a *bigger* behind."
> *Hans:* "Yes."
> *I:* "Like Daddy's; because you'd like to be Daddy."
> *Hans:* "Yes, and I'd like to have a moustache like yours and hairs like yours." (He pointed to the hairs on my chest.)

Instead of being made into a woman, the boy had been made into a grown man. He had assigned the plumber/doctor the task of completing what his "quite peculiarly lively interest in his wiwi-maker" had begun.[125]

The plumber had figured earlier in Hans's fantasy life. *"I was in the bath, and then the plumber came and unscrewed it. Then he took a big borer and stuck it into my stomach."* The meaning was not transparent, and here the father and Freud differed: the father thought that the two plumber fantasies meant the same thing; Freud interpreted this one as a fantasy of procreation "distorted by anxiety."

> The big bath of water, in which Hans imagined himself, was his mother's womb; the "borer," which his father had from the first recognized as a penis, owed its mention to its connection with "being born." The interpretation that we are obliged to give to the phantasy will of course sound very curious: "With your big penis you 'bored' me (i. e. "gave birth to me") and put me in my mother's womb."

When the boy first reported the fantasy, it had not been interpreted. It had "merely served Hans as a starting point from which to continue giving information"—and as it turned out, much of the information had to do with procreation.[126]

The boy, Freud wrote, was bound to approach that subject "by way of the excretory complex," and it came as no surprise that he should have expressed a "lively interest" in "lumf" (feces) as well as in wiwimakers. Up to this point the father had been out in front, and the boy "had merely followed his lead and come trotting after; but now it was Hans who was forging ahead, so rapidly and steadily that his father found it difficult to keep up with him." When his father did come abreast, he recognized the similarity between "a body loaded with faeces" and a heavily loaded cart, between the way feces left that body and the way a cart drove "out through a gateway." From the topic of lumf the boy moved on to that of his baby sister. The juxtaposition made interpretation easy: "Hanna was a lumf herself—. . . all babies were lumfs and born like lumfs."[127] Thus the heavily loaded carts, furniture-vans, and buses which frightened Hans symbolically represented pregnancy, and the falling horse which likewise frightened him represented his mother in childbirth.

Hans proceeded to be more explicit. With the aid of a doll he demonstrated how he imagined that birth took place. "He pushed a small penknife . . . in through a round hole in the body of an india-rubber doll, and then let it drop out again by tearing apart the doll's legs." At long last, the parents decided to enlighten their son—at least "up to a certain point." They told him that children grew inside their mothers and then were "brought into the world by being pressed out . . . like a 'lumf,'" and that that process involved a considerable amount of pain.[128]

What Hans refused to believe was that women alone could bear children. On this point his father had been explicit. "You know quite well that boys can't have children." Hans replied: "Well, yes. But I believe they can, all the same." Among the many children he imagined himself as having, the name of one "Lodi," which derived from a lumf-like sausage, led the father to ask a further question: "When you sat on the chamber[-pot] and a lumf came, did you think to yourself you were having a baby?" The boy answered, with delight, in the affirmative. In fantasy "he was a mother and wanted children with whom he could repeat the endearments that he himself had experienced." In this connection he urged his father to send the "Professor" (Freud) the following—the penultimate—report:

> "This morning I was in the W.C. with all my children. First I did lumf and wiwi-ed, and they looked on. Then I put them on the seat and they wiwi-ed and did lumf, and I wiped their behinds with paper. D'you know why? Because I'd so much like to have children; then I'd do everything for them—take them to the W.C., clean their behinds, and do everything that one does with children."

The message of Hans's fantasies was plain to tell:

> He was able to imagine the act of giving birth as a pleasurable one by relating it to his own first feelings of pleasure in passing stool; and he was thus able to find a double motive for wishing to have children of his own: the pleasure of giving birth to them and the pleasure . . . of looking after them.[129]

The message of the fantasy about the plumber giving him a bigger wiwi-maker had been equally plain. And in Hans's mind there was no conflict between the two messages: the erotogenic could endow the ego with more than one meaning.

.   .   .

"What can be more definite for a human being than what he has . . . felt on his own body?"[130] Daniel Paul Schreber posed this rhetorical question, and it was Schreber who represented the extreme case of the erotogenic fashioning an ego. With him, erotogenicity became separated from a privileged penis; with him, his self became increasingly female.

Daniel Paul Schreber had been born in 1842, the second son of the well-known orthopedist and educational reformer Daniel Gottlob Moritz Schreber. Trained in the law, the younger Schreber had a long and distinguished judicial career, chiefly in the kingdom of Saxony. Then, in October 1884, after an unsuccessful campaign for the Reichstag, he suffered his first breakdown and had to be hospitalized. The following June he was pronounced cured and received his discharge. For the next eight years all seemed well; he made further professional advances, becoming, in 1893, a presiding judge of Saxony's highest court. Those eight years, "rich" alike in the public and the private realm, were "marred only from time to time by the repeated disappointment" of his and his wife's hopes "of being blessed with children."[131] The period ended with a second breakdown, after which he was never again pronounced cured.

Dr. Weber, the superintendent of the Sonnenstein Asylum to which Schreber was transferred in 1894, and where he remained until 1902, described at some length "how out of the stormy tides . . . of acute insanity . . . a sediment was, so to speak, deposited and fixed, and gave the illness the picture of paranoia."[132] Those stormy tides stirred up hypochondriacal ideas: "he thought he was dead and rotten, suffering from the plague . . . that all sorts of horrible manipulations were being performed on his body"; they stirred up visual and auditory hallucinations to which at times he responded by "bellowing very loudly at the sun with threats and imprecations"; they caused eating disturbances: "he refused nourishment so that he had to be forcibly fed . . . [and] retained his stool, apparently deliberately"; and they caused sleep disturbances accompanied by such noisy behavior that for a number of months he had to be put in an isolated room. Gradually Schreber became accessible to those around him: he began to be able to control himself for short intervals; he "even answered simple questions about his condition." In the spring of 1897 a more marked change was observed: he "entered into a lively correspondence with his wife and other relatives; and . . . the letters were correctly and deftly written, and hardly showed anything pathological." He was, nevertheless, "filled with pathological ideas," which were "woven into a complete system, more or less fixed, and not amenable to correction by objective evidence."[133] And as one example of how such ideas in turn impaired Schreber's judgment, Dr. Weber cited the patient's wish to have his memoirs published.

In his preface Schreber explained why that had become an imperative:

> I started this work without having publication in mind. The idea only occurred to me as I progressed with it. . . . I believe that expert examination of my body and observation of my personal fate during my lifetime would be of value both for science and the knowledge of religious truths.

Even before he had entered into correspondence with his wife, Schreber had been putting down on paper "a few unconnected thoughts and words." From there he proceeded to keeping regular diaries; these he had written for his own benefit, assuming they would "remain beyond other people's comprehension."[134] Not so, he hoped, the memoirs, the bulk of which was composed in 1900. That same year he undertook legal steps for his release from tutelage (that is, guardianship by the courts), steps which in 1902 led to his discharge from the Sonnenstein Asylum. (In late 1907 he broke down again and remained in a mental institution until his death three and a half years later.) For the court the decisive issue was not whether Schreber was mentally ill—of that there was no doubt—but whether he was capable of taking care of his own affairs and defending his interests—of that the court seemed equally certain. Schreber's wish to publish his memoirs, Dr. Weber's testimony notwithstanding, had not told against him; in the eyes of the court that wish stood not as proof of incapacity to look out for himself but rather as proof "of the strength of his belief in the truth of the revelations which had been granted him by God."[135] In 1903 his wish was fulfilled. Having made substantial changes to his memoirs, Schreber saw them in print and brought "to the notice of a wider circle."[136] In that wider circle was Sigmund Freud.

In 1910 Freud took along with him on his summer holiday the memoirs of "the wonderful Schreber, who ought to have been made a professor of psychiatry and director of a mental hospital." During the following autumn he returned to them, and in the first part of December he put down on paper, in an essay entitled "Psycho-Analytic Notes on an Autobiographical Account of a Case of Paranoia," reflections prompted by the book. His own essay Freud described as "formally imperfect" and then, borrowing Schreber's vocabulary, as "fleetingly improvised." Still, he thought there were "a few good things in it," more particularly his boldest thrust yet at psychiatry: his theory of paranoia.[137]

Freud's interest in this disorder went back to the early stages of his investigations into psychopathology. It was part and parcel of his concern with the problem of the choice of neurosis. At the time he was writing about hysteria and postulating the mechanism of conversion to account for its symptoms, he was assigning to paranoia its own specific mechanism, that of projection.[138] His enthusiasm for linking paranoia and projection never waned; it was amply apparent in his essay on Schreber. So too was his zeal for fitting paranoia into his theory of psychosexual development. When at the end of the 1890s he had begun to see a connection between choice of neurosis and his sexual theory, he had made only a few cryptic remarks about how paranoia might be accommodated.[139] By the time he had read Schreber's memoirs he was ready to make up for past neglect; he was ready to discern in paranoia the projection (and distortion) of homosexual impulses.[140] No wonder, then, that Schreber's principal delusion, that of being transformed into a woman, riveted Freud's attention. (It should be noted that Freud offered no conceptual framework here for differentiating between the feminine and the homosexual.)[141]

A psychoanalyst, he wrote, should approach Schreber's delusional formations "with a suspicion that even thought-structures so extraordinary as these and so remote from our common modes of thinking" sprang from understandable "impulses of the human mind." The psychoanalyst would thus want to go "deeply into the details of the delusion and into the history of its development."[142] With these precepts to guide him, he set out to trace the vicissitudes of Schreber's "unmanning."

The initial bodily signs of being transformed into a woman, Schreber claimed, pointed to a plot laid against him.

> A conspiracy against me was brought to a head (in about March or April 1894). Its object was to contrive that, when once my nervous complaint had been recognized as incurable or assumed to be so, I should be handed over to a certain person in a particular manner: my soul was to be delivered up to him, but my body . . . was to be transformed into a female body, and as such surrendered to the person in question with a view to sexual abuse. . . .

It was not until later that "the idea forced itself" upon Schreber "that God Himself had played the part of accomplice, if not instigator, in the plot whereby" his "soul was to be murdered" and his "body used like a strumpet."[143]

But God did not prevail.

> Every attempt at murdering my soul, or at emasculating me for purposes *contrary to the Order of Things* (that is, for the gratification of the sexual appetites of a human individual), or later at destroying my understanding—every such attempt has come to nothing. From this apparently unequal struggle between one weak man and God Himself, I have emerged as the victor—though not without undergoing much bitter

suffering and privation—because the Order of Things stands upon my side.[144]

During the second round, so to speak, which began in November 1895, the signs of Schreber's unmanning became increasingly prominent and acquired a new meaning. Where heretofore the Order of Things had helped him resist emasculation, now that very Order "imperatively demanded" it.[145] In the event of a world catastrophe entailing the destruction of mankind—and Schreber was convinced that such a catastrophe had occurred—the Order required the survival of a single human being. Schreber was the one chosen. (For a long time he thought that all the others were merely "fleeting-improvised-men.")[146] And once he was chosen, the rest followed: he would be transformed into a woman, impregnated by divine rays, and give birth to a new race of men. It also followed that whether or not he personally liked it, there was no reasonable course open to him but to reconcile himself to this transformation.

Schreber's shorthand for the process was unmanning, and Freud echoed him in consistently referring to the delusion as one of emasculation—and a penis in retreat figured in the memoirs:

> Several times (particularly in bed) there were marked indications of an actual retraction of the male organ; . . . further the removal by miracles of single *hairs* from my *beard* and particularly my *moustache;* finally a *change in my whole stature* (diminution of body size)—probably due to a contraction of the vertebrae and possibly of my thigh bones.[147]

The unmanning included swelling breasts:

> When the [divine] rays approach, my breast gives the impression of a pretty well-developed female bosom; this phenomenon can be *seen* by anybody who wants to observe me *with his own eyes.* . . . A brief glance however would not suffice, the observer would have to go to the trouble of spending 10 or 15 minutes near me. In that way anybody would notice the periodic swelling and diminution of my bosom. Naturally hairs remain under my arms and on my chest; these are by the way sparse in my case; my nipples also remain small as in the male sex. Notwithstanding, I venture to assert flatly that anybody who sees me standing in front of a mirror with the upper part of my body naked would get the undoubted *impression of a female trunk*—especially when the illusion is strengthened by some feminine adornments.[148]

62

The medical examination to which Schreber was willing, indeed eager, to submit, would, he claimed, demonstrate that his femininity was something more than a matter of a retreating penis and swelling breasts. His whole body, he claimed, was "filled with nerves of voluptuousness" from head to foot, such as was "the case only in the adult female."

> When I exert light pressure with my hand on any part of my body I can *feel* certain string or cord-like structures under the skin; these are particularly marked on my chest where the woman's bosom is, here they have the peculiarity that one can feel them ending in nodular thickenings. Through pressure on one such structure I can produce a feeling of female sensuous pleasure, particularly if I think of something feminine. I do this, by the way, not for sensual lust, but I am absolutely compelled to do so if I want to achieve sleep or protect myself against otherwise unbearable pain.[149]

Schreber's body had thus acquired "the same susceptibility to stimulation" as was "possessed by the genitals."[150] According to Freud, it had become erotogenic; according to Schreber, its erotogenic quality little by little bestowed on him a feminine identity.

Schreber never finished the transformation that turned out to be far more complex than the shorthand metaphor of emasculation or castration would suggest.

> For several years . . . I lived in the certain expectation that one day my unmanning . . . would be completed . . . but whether . . . unmanning can really be completed I dare not predict. . . . It is therefore possible, indeed probable, that to the end of my days there will be strong indications of femaleness, but that I shall die a man.

In the meantime Schreber had "wholeheartedly inscribed the cultivation of femininity" on his "banner."[151] In the meantime he had demonstrated what Freud's notion of the erotogenic entailed, and what the founder of psychoanalysis at times forgot, that anatomy was not destiny.[152]

CHAPTER THREE

Redefining the Object

How does a subject come to know the object world? In the nineteenth century this question, or rather its Kantian formulation in terms of mind as a transcendental reality comprising elements or processes that made knowledge possible, became the overriding, indeed the defining, concern of professional philosophers. But it was not their concern alone. Psychologists could also lay claim to it. Ever since Locke, it had been a staple of psychological as well as philosophical discourse that understanding mental functioning went hand in hand with constructing a theory of knowledge. And as the nineteenth century drew to a close, psychologists made plain their intention of holding fast to this inheritance of epistemological worries.

Did Freud count himself among the legatees? In his late adolescence, more particularly during his second year at the University of Vienna, he ruminated about problems of this sort. On November 8, 1874, he wrote his friend Eduard Silberstein that he, a "godless medical man and empiricist," was "attending two courses in philosophy." One of them was taught by the ex-priest Franz Brentano, and Freud's letters during the academic year 1874–75 attest to the profound impression Brentano was making on him—even to the point of inducing him to question, albeit temporarily, his own godlessness. He was not, however, induced to question his empiricism. Quite the contrary: his teacher too, Freud wrote, "declared himself unreservedly a follower of the empiricist school" and accordingly advocated applying "the method of science to philosophy and to psychology."[1] (Hume ranked highest in Brentano's pantheon. He regarded the Scot as "the most precise thinker and most perfect writer of all philosophers," and what people praised in Kant he credited to Hume. What was "entirely Kant's own he rejected as harmful and untrue." As for Schelling, Fichte, and Hegel, he dismissed them as "swindlers.")[2] By March 1875, with Brentano's encouragement, Freud had decided to combine his medical studies with philosophy, to attend two faculties and acquire two doctorates. It was a plan he soon abandoned. Six months later, after his first visit to the homeland of his current favorites, "Tyndall, Huxley, Lyell, Darwin," he wrote that he was now "more suspicious than ever of philosophy."[3]

Did he remain in that frame of mind? On January 1, 1896, he wrote to Wilhelm Fliess that he secretly nourished the "hope of arriving," via "the detour of medical practice," at his "initial goal of philosophy." Four years later he reported that he had "just acquired Nietzsche" but had "not opened him yet." He was "too lazy."[4] (Subsequently he claimed that as a young man he had had little "taste for reading philosophical works.")[5] In this same letter Freud penned his famous self-portrait: he was "not at all a man of science, not an observer, not an experimenter, not a thinker. . . . By temperament" he was "nothing but a conquistador . . . with all the curiosity, daring, and tenacity characteristic of a man of this sort."[6] From such conflicting statements one might well conclude that tracking Freud's interest or lack of interest in philosophical problems in general and epistemology in particular is not rewarding.[7]

Still, traditional epistemological concerns managed to insinuate themselves. How could it be otherwise, once Freud had located the origin of his patients' neurotic suffering in their earliest years? He introduced the object world of childhood into the unconscious domain and then offered an account of how that world was distorted. When he shifted his attention from the object world to the ego as object, he also gave the subject-object problem a new (revolutionary?) twist: it became a matter of experiences with an object world already distorted, altering the ego (once again understood as self).[8]

"Relics of Antiquity"

In his paper entitled "Screen Memories" (1899) Freud drew upon his own recollections (thinly disguised)[9] to explore why certain childhood scenes, which in themselves appeared of little significance, became fixed in memory. Among them he singled out "one . . . long scene":

> I see a rectangular, rather steeply sloping piece of meadow-land, green and thickly grown; in the green there are a great number of yellow flowers—evidently common dandelions. At the top end of the meadow there is a cottage and in front of the cottage-door two women are standing chatting busily, a peasant-woman with a handkerchief on her head and a children's nurse. Three children are playing in the grass. One of them is myself (between the age of two and three); the two others are my boy cousin, who is a year older than me, and his sister, who is almost exactly the same age as I am. We are picking the yellow flowers and each of us is holding a bunch of flowers we have already picked. The little girl has the best bunch; and, as though by mutual agreement, we—the two boys—fall on her and snatch away her flowers. She runs up the meadow in tears and as a consolation the peasant-woman gives her a big piece of black bread. Hardly have we seen this than we throw the flowers away, hurry to the cottage and ask to be given some bread too. And we are in fact given some. . . . In my memory the bread tastes quite delicious—and at that point the scene breaks off.[10]

The impressions of those childhood years had been stirred up on two subsequent occasions, which Freud proceeded to narrate. On the first one he had just turned seventeen. That summer he revisited his birthplace, Freiberg (now Příbor) in Moravia. Economic catastrophe, the collapse of his father's "branch of industry," had forced his family to move more than fourteen years earlier. "Long and difficult years followed, of which . . . nothing was worth remembering." When Freud finally returned, alone, he stayed with old friends of his parents, who in the intervening years had "risen greatly in the world." He found the contrast painful between their rural comfort and his own family's straitened circumstances in an urban environment he disliked. What was more important, his hosts had an attractive young daughter, aged fifteen, with whom Freud "immediately fell in love." It was his "first calf-love and sufficiently intense." When the girl left for school, his "longings" reached "a really high pitch"—and with them came a flood of regrets.[11] He bemoaned the fact that his family's prospects had been blighted, that he had been deprived of the chance to grow up where he had been born, to find and follow a path marked out by his father, and, above all, to marry the lovely young creature.

67

The second occasion dated from three years later. During his summer holiday Freud visited his "uncle" (actually his older half-brother) and met again the two children who appeared in the "childhood scene with the dandelions." This family too had left Freiberg, at the same time as his, and unlike his own, had prospered in their new location (actually Manchester). By the summer Freud visited them, he had become a student at the University and had also become such a "slave" to his books that he had "had nothing left over" for his "cousin" (actually his niece). This time there had been no falling in love, and no marital fancies had danced in his head. His father and his "uncle," however, had entertained thoughts along those lines, and later so did Freud, after he became "a newly-fledged man of science . . . hard pressed by the exigencies of life." Then he had sometimes "reflected" that "his father had meant well in planning such a marriage for him."[12]

Freud was on his way to answering his question about what got remembered. It was probable that he had amalgamated hopes and aspirations from the two occasions with one another and "made a childhood memory of them." The features that linked up with the second occasion were the easier to detect. The principal actors were identical, and a principal, if not the principal, action, "throwing away the flowers in exchange for bread," struck Freud "as not a bad disguise" for the marriage plan his father had entertained: he was to give up his "unpractical ideals and take on a 'bread-and-butter' occupation." The flavor of the bread itself, which seemed to him "exaggerated in an almost hallucinatory fashion," summoned up the first occasion: it brought back his musings about "how sweet the bread would have tasted" had he married the lovely young creature. The recollected yellow of the dandelions, whose clarity and vividness were also exaggerated, linked up with the actual girl. The first time Freud had met her, she was wearing a yellow dress and the color made a deep impression on him; but it was yellowish brown, "more like the colour of wallflowers" than that of dandelions. Here a third occasion, that of seeing certain Alpine flowers which had "light colouring in the lowlands" and "darker shades at higher altitudes," made a contribution. When Freud had been struggling for his "daily bread," mountaineering had been the one enjoyment he had allowed himself, and through this indulgence he had become acquainted with the Alps.[13] These Alpine flowers thus served as a "stamp giving the date" at which the childhood scene had been recalled. Thereafter it had remained fixed in Freud's memory.

What moral did he draw from the tale? The more obvious was to cast doubt on the historical accuracy of recollection. "The isolated childhood memories," he commented, "that people have possessed consciously from time immemorial and before there was any such thing as analysis" might have been "falsified" or at least might "combine truth and falsehood in plenty."[14] It might be more appropriate, after all, to conclude that his own specimen memory had been manufactured, like a work of fiction, rather than to suppose that it had emerged. In short, there was "no guarantee of the data produced by . . . memory."[15]

That the childhood scene might not have occurred—or have occurred in some fashion other than the one consciously remembered—did not deter Freud from drawing a second, and far less obvious, conclusion from his specimen, which he named a "screen memory." Its value, he argued, lay not in its content, but in "the relation existing between that content and some other" that had been excluded from consciousness.[16] (Freud uncovered a sexual wish, "to deflower," represented by "taking away flowers from a girl," which, in 1899, he ascribed to adolescence.)[17] A decade and a half later, in his essay "Remembering, Repeating and Working-Through," Freud expressed more forcefully what he regarded as the real worth of screen memories:

> Forgetting impressions, scenes or experiences nearly always reduces itself to shutting them off. . . . "Forgetting" [however] becomes . . . restricted when we assess at their true value the screen memories which are so generally present. In some cases I have had the impression that the familiar childhood amnesia . . . is completely counterbalanced by screen memories. Not only *some* but *all* of what is essential from childhood has been retained in these memories. It is simply a question of knowing how to extract it out of them by analysis.[18]

.   .   .

Screen memories promised to compensate for childhood amnesia. So did dreams. They reproduced material from childhood; they had at their command material from childhood which for the most part had been blotted out by gaps in conscious memory. Authorities on dreaming, authorities Freud referred to in his review of the literature, had frequently drawn attention to these facts.[19]

In that literature the example he seemed to prefer—he cited it twice—was reported by L. F. A. Maury in his *Le sommeil et les rêves*.

> It was dreamt by a Monsieur F., who as a child had lived at Montbrison. Twenty-five years after leaving it, he decided to revisit his home and some friends of the family whom he had not since met. During the night before his departure he dreamt that he was already at Montbrison and . . . met a gentleman whom he did not know by sight but who told him he was Monsieur T., a friend of his father's.

On waking, Monsieur F. recalled that he had once known someone by that name but had no recollection of what the man looked like. "A few days later he actually reached Montbrison, . . . and there met a gentleman whom he at once recognized as the Monsieur T. in the dream. The real person, however, looked much older."[20] The accuracy of the childhood memory emerging in the dream had received a dramatic confirmation.

Freud had a similar experience of his own to recount. He had dreamt of someone who, in the dream, he knew had been the doctor in his native town. Yet the face was indistinct; it was "confused with a picture" of one of his secondary school teachers.[21] Why the confusion? In this case it was not a visual image of a man, but a connection between two men that was emerging in the dream. Left to himself, Freud was unable to identify the connection. He turned to his mother, and she cleared up the mystery: she told him that his childhood doctor "had only one eye," and of all Freud's schoolteachers only the one that showed up in the dream had "the same defect."[22]

The dream Maury reported Freud interpreted as signifying impatience: the dreamer wished to go to Montbrison and in his impatience had fulfilled his wish by dreaming himself already there. His own dream Freud did not fully interpret. In the 1909 edition of *The Interpretation of Dreams* he added that he had not seen the doctor since the age of three, and as far as he remembered had not thought of him in waking life. He bore, however, a scar on his chin—the result of an accident—which could have reminded him of the doctor's ministrations.[23] In that same edition Freud also added, in the context of discussing examination dreams, further information about the schoolteacher, with whom Freud had had a very comfortable, indeed conspiratorial, relationship:

> In my dreams of school examinations, I am invariably examined in History, in which I did brilliantly—though only, it is true, because . . . my kindly master . . . did not fail to notice that on the paper of questions which I handed him back I had run my finger-nail through the middle one of the three questions included, to warn him not to insist upon that particular one.[24]

It was when he began tracking experiences of this sort, experiences belonging to a dream's latent rather than to its manifest content, that Freud expected to recover the richest material.

This was true of a series of dreams based on his passionate desire to visit Rome. (He did not fulfill that wish in waking life until the summer of 1901. In the meantime he satisfied in his dream life a "longing for Rome" which he regarded as "deeply neurotic.")[25] Five summers earlier he and his younger brother Alexander had gotten within fifty miles of the Eternal City, and in December of that year he had proposed to Fliess that they hold a "congress on Italian soil! (Naples, Pompeii)." Apparently Fliess suggested that they meet in Prague instead, and eventually the meeting took place in Nuremberg in the spring of the following year. The prospect of a "congress" in Prague prompted the fourth of the dream series. On the dream-day Freud had written to Fliess to say that "Prague might not be an agreeable place for a German to walk about in." As for the dream itself, it was nothing more than setting and signs: "It took me to Rome once more. I saw a street-corner before me and was surprised to find so many posters in German stuck up there."[26] When Freud awoke, as he reported to Fliess, he "immediately thought: so this was Prague" and recalled a wish, probably dating from his "student days, that the German language might be better tolerated" there by the Czech-speaking majority.[27]

The theme of bilingualism had a double aspect. Latin and German, the two principal languages in Freud's secondary school education, figured in the dream's manifest content—he was surprised at the absence of Latin inscriptions and the presence of German posters. Czech and German, the languages of Freud's earliest years, appeared in its latent content. The dream reminded him of Czech, which he was certain he had understood as an infant, and of a nursery rhyme in that language, which he had heard during his adolescent visit to Freiberg, had learned with great ease, and still knew by heart, without, however, having any idea what it meant. Just as the "ancient" languages, in this case Czech as well as Latin, had not been obliterated and could still be revived, so too repressed memories might return.[28]

And so one did—a powerful one. In a memory concerning his father that dated from late childhood, Freud located the common source of the four "Rome" dreams. (Jacob Freud had died in October 1896, and at the time of the dream, his son was still mourning his loss.)

> I may have been ten or twelve years old, when my father began to take me with him on his walks and reveal to me in his talk his views upon things in the world we live in. Thus it was, on one such occasion, that he told me a story to show me how much better things were now than they had been in his days. "When I was a young man," he said, "I went for a walk one Saturday in the streets of your birthplace, I was well dressed, and had a new fur cap on my head. A Christian came up to me and with a single blow knocked off my cap into the mud and shouted: 'Jew! get off the pavement!'" "And what did you do?" I asked. "I went into the roadway and picked up my cap," was his quiet reply. This struck me as unheroic conduct on the part of the big, strong man who was holding the little boy by the hand.[29]

Thinking on Rome, prompted to do so by the manifest content of the dream, Freud recalled that his journey of the previous summer had taken him close to Rome, "past Lake Trasimene," but no farther:

> I had . . . been following in Hannibal's footsteps. Like him, I had been fated not to see Rome. . . . But Hannibal . . . had been the favorite hero of my later school days. Like so many boys of that age, I had sympathized in the Punic Wars not with the Romans but with the Carthaginians. And when in the higher classes I began to understand for the first time what it meant to belong to an alien race, and anti-semitic feelings among the other boys warned me that I must take up a definite position, the figure of the semitic general rose still higher in my esteem. To my youthful mind Hannibal and Rome symbolized the conflict between the tenacity of Jewry and the organization of the Catholic church.

Jacob Freud suffered by comparison: "I contrasted . . . [my father's] situation with another which fitted my feelings better: the scene in which Hannibal's father, Hamilcar Barca, made his boy swear before the household altar to take vengeance on the Romans."[30]

In the first edition of *The Interpretation of Dreams,* Freud had misidentified Hannibal's father; he had called him Hasdrubal, which was "the name of Hannibal's *brother,* as well as of his brother-in-law and predecessor in command." The error "annoyed" Freud; it also turned out to be grist for his mill, that is, to provide further evidence on which to test his notion that errors of memory should be regarded as distortions "rooted in repressed material" or, as in this instance, suppressed material.[31] (Errors expressed a range of intentions that had in common having been in some way "forced back.")[32] In this instance Freud had intended to be discreet: he had intended to conceal further reflections or musings prompted by the memory of his father, musings which were known to him and which he subsequently revealed in *The Psychopathology of Everyday Life.*

> I could have gone on to tell how my relationship with my father was changed by a visit to England, which resulted in my getting to know my half-brother. . . . [Suppressed] phantasies of how different things would have been if I had been born the son not of my father but of my brother . . . falsified the text of my book at the place where I broke off the analysis, by forcing me to put the brother's name for the father's.[33]

Thus the error had betrayed the train of thought Freud had wanted to conceal.

Once again, as with screen memories, conscious or preconscious memory had proved fallible. What guarantee, then, could there be that unconscious memories derived from dreams were free from error or distortion? Freud's answer mixed caution and audacity. Whether the memory was represented fully in a dream's manifest content or was merely alluded to and arrived at in the course of interpreting the dream, "proof" that what had emerged were actually "impressions from childhood" could "be established" only by referring to "external evidence," and there was "seldom an opportunity for doing this." Yet the absence of such evidence did not deter Freud. "A whole number of factors in psychoanalytic work," which were "mutually consistent" and thus seemed "sufficiently trustworthy," provided a "general justification for inferring . . . childhood experiences from dreams."[34] At the outset, the analyst might be in doubt whether he was "dealing with reality"; later "certain indications" would enable him to come to a decision.[35] Freud's confidence about uncovering the historical past was not easily shaken.

.   .   .

> There is not only *method* in madness, as the poet had already perceived, but also a fragment of *historical* truth.[36]
> Psychiatric delusions . . . contain a small fragment of truth and the patient's conviction extends over from this truth on to its delusional wrappings.[37]

These words, penned near the end of Freud's long life, were simply the last of a series of such aphorisms scattered throughout his corpus.[38] At the same time he fastened on the metaphor of analytic work as archeology and the analyst as archeologist. It turned up in the preface to his case history "Fragment of an Analysis":

> In face of the incompleteness of my analytic results, I had no choice but to follow the example of those discoverers whose good fortune it is to bring to the light of day after their long burial the priceless though mutilated relics of antiquity. I have restored what is missing, taking the best models known to me from other analyses; but, like a conscientious archaeologist, I have not omitted to mention in each case where the authentic parts end and my constructions begin.[39]

More than a figure of speech was involved. Freud's passion for collecting "relics of antiquity," a passion which in his middle years he increasingly indulged, led one patient to comment that his rooms "in no way reminded one of a doctor's office but rather of an archeologist's study."[40] Poetry, delusions, and archeology all came together in Wilhelm Jensen's *Gradiva*. Freud could not fail to have been captivated.

In the world's estimation *Gradiva*, first published in 1903, ranked as a minor novella and its author as a minor German playwright and novelist. Freud did not dispute these rankings but only that *Gradiva* should be regarded as mere fancy. In general, he viewed creative writers as "valuable allies," who were "apt to know a whole host of things between heaven and earth" of which his "philosophy" had not yet begun to "dream." And in particular, he considered Jensen's "descriptions . . . so faithfully copied from reality" that it would be fully appropriate to treat the work, if not precisely as "a psychiatric study," at least as offering evidence for such a study.[41] Freud did just that in the analysis of the novella he published in 1907.

The protagonist, Norbert Hanold, was a young archeologist. So absorbed in his academic pursuits had he become that he "had turned completely from life and its pleasures." He cared more about marble and bronze than he did about flesh and blood. But a "corrective" was at work: he had been endowed with "an extremely lively imagination . . . of an entirely unscientific sort."[42] And on a trip to Rome, in a museum of antiquities, he had found an object for that imagination to dwell on. It was a relief, a plaster cast of which he hung in his room so that he might continually gaze upon it. His fascination with the sculpture was the psychological starting point of the narrative.

The relief "represented a fully-grown girl . . . with her flowing dress a little pulled up so as to reveal her sandalled feet. One foot rested squarely on the ground; the other, lifted from the ground in the act of following after, touched it only with the tips of the toes, while the sole and heel rose almost perpendicularly"[43] This charming and peculiar gait riveted Hanold's attention, and he gave the young woman a Latinate name, "Gradiva"—"the girl who steps along."[44] It also puzzled him. Had the sculptor, he wondered, copied it from nature? He determined to find out: "in dry, but more especially in wet, weather," he took to examining "women's and girls' feet as they came into view—an activity which brought him some angry, and some encouraging, glances" from those he thus observed.[45] No one, he concluded, had the gait he sought. Still he found "something of today" about "Gradiva."[46]

His "scientific" investigations had reached a dead end; his imaginative pursuit took off. First in waking life and then in sleep, he became convinced that she had been a native of Pompeii. And there, in a terrifying dream, he saw himself also, on the very day Vesuvius erupted. Suddenly he spied Gradiva; he tried to warn her of what might befall her; she, calmly stepping along, continued on her way to a temple, where she took a "seat on one of the steps and slowly laid her head down on it, while her face grew paler and paler, as though it were turning to marble." She remained, "like someone asleep, till the rain of ashes buried her form." Hanold awoke with "the confused shouts of the inhabitants of Pompeii" echoing in his ears.[47] The dream itself continued to reverberate; it transformed Hanold's fantasy about Gradiva's life and death into a delusion.

And so he resolved "to make a spring-time journey to Italy."[48] He acted on impulse, "from a feeling he could not name."[49] "An inner restlessness and dissatisfaction drove him from Rome to Naples and from thence" to Pompeii.[50] But he had no glimmer of what he was seeking. It had not dawned on him that he had started on his travels "in order to see whether he could find any traces" of "Gradiva."[51] He discovered more than a trace; he discovered a living embodiment.

The first meeting took place at mid-day. Suddenly Hanold saw the young woman of his relief emerge from a house and tread lightly over lava stepping-stones to the other side of the street, just as he had seen her do in his dream. He followed after and found her sitting on some low stones. He addressed her in Greek—though he assumed she was a native of Pompeii, he had initially discerned something Hellenic about her; she gave no answer. Then he addressed her in Latin; again no response. Finally, with a smile playing about her lips: "If you want to speak to me," she said, "you must do it in German."[52] But Hanold was not to be "torn from his delusion." He thought "Gradiva" was a mid-day ghost—the ancients regarded noon as the hour at which ghosts returned fleetingly; and when a pretty butterfly fluttered around her before she slipped away, he interpreted it "as a messenger from Hades reminding the dead girl that . . . the . . . hour . . . was at an end."[53] Her knowledge of the German language should have struck him as odd—still more, his own exclamation: "I knew your voice sounded like that."[54] Hanold, presumably, had never heard it, not even in his dream. He made only one further remark to her—a request that she come again the next day at the same time and to the same place.

The following day she reappeared, ready to enter into Hanold's delusion and yet determined in due course to free him from it. She elicited its "whole compass . . . without ever contradicting it . . . she learnt of his dream, in which she had perished along with her native city, and then of the marble relief and the posture of the foot which had so much attracted the archaeologist." And when she prepared to demonstrate her gait, she took care to explain that as "an adaptation to the present day," instead of sandals she was wearing "light-sand-coloured shoes of fine leather."[55] And she gave him her name, Zoë. It rang no bells with Hanold; he had no inkling of why the relief, as well as Zoë herself, had "something of today" about them.

When she reappeared on the following day, the reality of her presence began to shake Hanold's delusion. He started to exercise his reason and to suspect that Zoë-Gradiva was something other than a mid-day ghost. He determined to experiment: in pursuit of a fly, he managed to slap her hand and discovered that "he had without any doubt touched . . . real, living, warm human" flesh. His delight was brief. When Zoë burst out with "There's no doubt you're out of your mind, Norbert Hanold!"[56] he took fright and fled, aware at last that he had been laboring under a misapprehension. But if not with a young Pompeian woman, with whom, he wondered, had he been associating? The answer lay beyond his power of ratiocination.

Zoë caught up with the bewildered young man, who jabbered about how inexplicable it was that she should have known his name. She revealed that she was in reality Fräulein Bertgang, a very close neighbor of his, and hence "knew him by sight and by name."[57] Had that been the entire explanation, Freud, for one, would have been disappointed. He expected more, and more was forthcoming. (So long as Hanold had thought Zoë a mid-day ghost who somehow knew German, he had used the familiar "du" form. When he realized his mistake and came to see her as a living creature, he had shifted to the formal "Sie." For Zoë the "du" remained the more natural, and she had ample justification for thinking so.) It turned out that as children she and Hanold had "run about together in a friendly way or sometimes . . . used to bump and thump each other." In the intervening years, archeology had taken hold of Hanold, and he, so Zoë told him, had "become an unbearable person who . . . no longer had any eyes in his head or tongue in his mouth," or memory of their early romance.[58] Zoë's work was nearly complete—living happily ever after was on the couple's horizon. Freud's remained to be done.

He proceeded to write of Hanold "as someone in real life." Accordingly he argued that the young archeologist's fantasies "were not capricious products of his imagination, but determined, without his knowing it, by the store of childhood impressions which he had forgotten, but which were still at work in him." Behind the marble relief, "the living Zoë whom he had neglected made her influence felt."[59] That influence (and their childhood relationship) accounted for all sorts of odd or ambiguous happenings in their Pompeiian conversations. It also explained the name. "Gradiva" was a translation of Zoë's surname, Bertgang: both signified someone "who steps along brilliantly."[60] Zoë herself, Freud concluded, shared his view of Hanold's delusion as "transformed memories"; from the outset she had recognized that "his interest in Gradiva had related" to her own person, and that it betokened the survival of his earlier affection.[61] Herein lay a fragment of historical truth.

. . .

On September 21, 1897, Freud had written Fliess confiding the "great secret" that in "the last few months" had been "slowly dawning": he no longer believed in his *"neurotica,"* that is, his theory of the defense neuroses.[62] The theory in question, which had made its debut in print the previous year, postulated a sexual etiology for hysteria and for obsessions as well.[63] (Freud had already designated current sexual practices as the causal agent in the actual neuroses—neurasthenia and anxiety neurosis.) For the defense neuroses he had assigned the causal role to a sexual experience in early childhood, by which he meant before puberty. Though he stipulated a different experience for each neurosis, he had loosely grouped them together under the label "seduction," and the theory became known as the seduction hypothesis. Now he expressed doubts, at least in part because "in the most deep-reaching psychosis . . . the secret of childhood experiences" was "not disclosed . . . the unconscious never" completely overcame "the resistance of the conscious."[64]

In framing the seduction hypothesis, Freud had invited history, and along with it the object world, into the unconscious domain; in retreating from that hypothesis he had no intention of rescinding his invitation.[65] Historical reality might be difficult to uncover; but with screen memories, dreams, and even delusions at his disposal, he was determined to continue his archeological quest.

Creations of Fantasy

When Freud wrote up Dora's case history, he conceived of it as a supplement to *The Interpretation of Dreams*. And he expected his readers to be familiar with that work; if they were not, they would, he predicted, "find only bewilderment . . . instead of . . . enlightenment" and would "certainly be inclined" to blame "the author and pronounce his views fantastic."[66] At the same time Freud expected his audience to be familiar with his and Breuer's *Studies on Hysteria* and his paper "The Aetiology of Hysteria," that is, to be conversant with the notion of psychical trauma in general and that of the traumatic nature of infantile or childhood sexual scenes in particular—in short, the seduction hypothesis. At the time he published Dora's case history, Freud did not admit publicly—he was to do so a year later—that he was no longer convinced of his own theory. He thus found himself in the awkward position of contriving a new etiology without formally discarding the old. The requirements of the new formulation were quite definite: it had to originate in childhood; it had to implicate sexuality (but not seduction); and it had to point to an explanation of his earlier error.

To accomplish his task Freud exploited material that turned up in a dream. The dream, "a periodically recurrent" one, was "well calculated to arouse" his "curiosity."[67] He had earlier commented that when "a dream was first dreamt in childhood" and then reappeared "from time to time during adult sleep," one could be sure that experiences of childhood would surface in its manifest content.[68] Here is the dream Dora reported:

> *A house was on fire. My father was standing beside my bed and woke me up. I dressed quickly. Mother wanted to stop and save her jewel-case; but Father said: "I refuse to let myself and my two children be burnt for the sake of your jewel-case." We hurried downstairs, and as soon as I was outside I woke up.*[69]

Freud asked his patient "to take the dream bit by bit" and to tell him "what occurred in connection" with different bits. Something quite recent came to Dora's mind:

> Father has been having a dispute with Mother in the last few days, because she locks the dining-room door at night. My brother's room, you see, has no separate entrance, but can only be reached through the dining room. Father does not want my brother to be locked in like that at night.[70]

Dora now remembered instances of dreaming the dream two years earlier, at the time of the second scene with Herr K.—the scene by the lake. Under Freud's prodding, Dora vouchsafed "hitherto forgotten details" about the events which had taken place there.[71] She recalled, after being propositioned, having a nap and waking from it to find Herr K. standing beside her bed as her father had done in the dream; the following morning, locking herself in—and Herr K. out—in order to dress, and dressing quickly; that afternoon discovering the key gone; and finally making a resolution to flee from the spot with her father. Each night, until that intention was carried out, the dream recurred. (Freud's interpretation of the jewel-case fitted in here: "jewel-case" turned out to be a "favourite expression . . . for the female genitals.")[72]

Something from childhood, he was convinced, had appeared in the manifest content. But which element captured a childhood scene? With this question in mind, Freud returned to Dora's first association to the dream. Her father, she had said, objected to her mother's locking the dining room door by remarking: "something might happen in the night so that it might be necessary to leave the room." The words had taken Freud aback and prompted him to interpret:

> Surely the allusion must be to a physical need: And if you transpose the accident into childhood what can it be but bed-wetting? But what is usually done to prevent children from wetting their bed? Are they not woken up in the night out of their sleep, *exactly as your father woke you up in the dream?* This, then, must be the actual occurrence which enabled you to substitute your father for Herr. K., who really woke you up out of your sleep. I am accordingly driven to conclude that you were addicted to bed-wetting up to a later age than is usual with children. The same must also have been true of your brother; for your father said: "*I refuse to let my two children* go to their destruction."[73]

Her brother, Dora acknowledged, had wetted his bed up to the age of six or seven. As for herself, she initially demurred, but on further reflection recalled that when she was seven or eight, she too had suffered in a similar fashion. With enuresis now an established fact, Freud was ready to take up the matter of etiology.

"During the years of childhood," he was to comment in the *Three Essays*, "most of the so-called bladder disturbances" were "sexual disturbances: nocturnal enuresis" corresponded to "a nocturnal emission."[74] According to this view, bed-wetting was a sign of sexual excitation; so too was masturbation. In writing up Dora's case history, Freud claimed more bluntly that, to the best of his knowledge, bed-wetting was caused by masturbation. Here what had been garnered from the dream fitted in with "a line of enquiry" Freud and Dora had been pursuing at that juncture—one that "led straight towards an admission that she had masturbated in childhood." It was an admission she never made, at least not in so many words; she "denied flatly that she could remember any such thing."

> But a few days later she did something which I [Freud] could not help regarding as a further step towards the confession. For on that day she wore at her waist—a thing she never did on any other occasion before or after—a small reticule of a shape which had just come into fashion; and, as she lay on the sofa and talked, she kept playing with it—opening it, putting a finger into it, shutting it again, and so on. I looked on for some time and then explained to her the nature of a "symptomatic act."[75]

Shortly before, Dora herself had raised the question of why she had fallen ill. Freud, now certain of her masturbatory history, gave an unequivocal answer: her hysterical symptoms had set in *after* she had stopped masturbating, and they provided a substitute satisfaction.[76]

At this point those readers familiar with his writings on the defense neuroses might well have felt perplexed. Those familiar with his writings on the actual neuroses might have fared better. Without fully acknowledging it, Freud found himself borrowing sexual abstinence from anxiety neurosis, pushing it back to childhood, and then offering it in an etiological account of a defense neurosis. In this fashion he had begun to contrive a new etiology that belonged to childhood and implicated sexuality, but he had not yet begun to suggest an explanation of why hysterical patients had so frequently reported seduction.

Freud's own version of how he came to such an explanation oversimplified a complicated process:

> When this etiology [seduction] broke down . . . , the result at first was helpless bewilderment. . . . At last came the reflection that, after all, one had no right to despair because one had been deceived in one's expectations; one must revise those expectations. If hysterical subjects trace back their symptoms to traumas that are fictitious, then the new fact which emerges is precisely that they create such scenes in *phantasy.*[77]

In fact it took Freud roughly a decade to replace experiences of seduction with fantasies thereof. And masturbation served as his point of departure.

In 1910 masturbation and masturbatory fantasies were the subject of three meetings of the Vienna Psychoanalytic Society (sucessor to the Wednesday Psychological Society), and in late 1911 and early 1912 they were discussed at an additional series of nine.[78] On the evening of January 24, 1912, the discussion centered on the difficulty of gathering reliable information about childhood masturbation from adult patients. It was at this point that Freud offered his clearest explanation of the role masturbation had played.

> Since childhood masturbation is such a general occurrence and is at the same time so poorly remembered, it must have an equivalent in psychic life. And, in fact, it is found in the fantasy encountered in most female patients—namely, that the father seduced her in childhood. This is the later reworking which is designed to cover up the recollection of infantile sexual activity and represents an excuse and an extenuation thereof. The grain of truth contained in this fantasy lies in the fact that the father, by way of his innocent caresses in earliest childhood, has actually awakened the little girl's sexuality (the same thing applies to the little boy and his mother). It is these same affectionate fathers that are the ones who then endeavor to break the child of the habit of masturbation, of which they themselves had by that time become the unwitting cause. And thus the motifs mingle in the most successful fashion to form this fantasy, which often dominates a woman's entire life (seduction fantasy): one part truth, one part gratification of love, and one part revenge.[79]

Masturbation itself, Freud argued, was a compound of "active behaviour" and "evocation of phantasy," and to describe that compound he employed the metaphor of soldering together—"*Verlötung.*"[80] The metaphor called to mind his notion that sexuality too was a compound: in his paper on anxiety neurosis he had outlined his conception of sexuality as psychosexual and had postulated a linkage between somatic sexual excitation and psychical desire; in 1897 he had written Fliess that impulses and fantasies were sometimes "put together";[81] and in the *Three Essays* he had posited a distinction between aim and object (understood as persons or parts of persons) and had described them as merely "soldered together."[82] His compounds, viewed in sequence, pointed to the next step, one that ranked as crucial: the soldering together of object and sexually saturated fantasy—and therewith a new etiology.

.   .   .

Oedipus had already made a public appearance, albeit without much fanfare, in *The Interpretation of Dreams*. He had turned up in a section devoted to typical dreams, under which rubric Freud had fitted dreams of the death of parents. Such dreams expressed in unusually direct fashion—and Freud took pains to try to explain that directness[83]—death-wishes preponderantly toward the parent of the same sex as the dreamer: that is, men dreamed "most frequently of their father's death and women of their mother's."[84]

How to account for this violation of "the cultural standards of filial piety"? Freud proposed a simple answer: children had wishes; parents blocked them; hostility ensued. The wishes singled out were the child's "first stirrings of sexuality." Freud had already learned from neurotics—and in this respect they did not "differ sharply . . . from other human beings"—that a child's sexual wishes awakened very early; that a "girl's first affection" was for her father and a "boy's first childish desires" were for his mother; and that the parent of the same sex figured as a "disturbing rival." (It took Freud another quarter-century to appreciate that a girl's first affection was for her mother.)[85] He continued:

> A particularly gifted and lively girl of four, in whom this piece of child psychology is especially transparent, declared quite openly: "Mummy can go away now. Then Daddy must marry me and I'll be his wife." . . . If a little boy is allowed to sleep beside his mother when his father is away from home, but has to go back to the nursery . . . as soon as his father returns, he may easily begin to form a wish that his father should *always* be away, so that he himself could keep his place beside his dear, lovely Mummy. One obvious way of attaining this wish would be if his father were dead; for the child has learnt one thing by experience—namely that "dead" people, such as Grandaddy, are always away and never come back.[86]

Freud then interpolated—or associated to—Sophocles' drama of *Oedipus Rex*.

> At a point when Oedipus, though he is not yet enlightened, has begun to feel troubled . . . Jocasta consoles him by referring to a dream which many people dream, though, as she thinks, it has no meaning: "Many a man ere now in dreams hath lain / With her who bore him." To-day, just as then, many men dream of having sexual relations with their

mothers, and speak of the fact with indignation and astonishment. It is clearly the key to the tragedy and the complement to the dream of the dreamer's father being dead.[87]

Here was a second typical dream that dovetailed with the first (the death of parents), just as love of the opposite-sex parent dovetailed with hostility to the parent of the same sex. A third dream remained concealed: a dream of parental revenge. In Freud's reading of the oedipal legend, the son's fear of his father's retaliation figured as central. (The Greek tragic hero was actually the victim of a preemptive strike. "Oedipus, son of Laïus, king of Thebes, and of Jocasta," Freud noted, "was exposed as an infant because an oracle had warned Laïus that the still unborn child would be his father's murderer.")[88]

Almost a decade later, Freud encountered a little Oedipus in Little Hans. The boy's attitude toward his father and mother confirmed "in the most concrete and uncompromising manner" what he had said in *The Interpretation of Dreams.* And when Hans had visited him, Freud had interpreted his difficulties along those lines: fondness for his mother; hostility toward his father; fear of his father; and finally the connection between father and horse. His father, Freud told the boy, was not really angry with him—despite his loving his mother so much—and "he might admit everything to him without any fear."[89]

In writing up the story of Hans's phobia, Freud had not been intent on finding support for the *The Interpretation of Dreams;* his concern, after all, was whether the picture drawn of the boy's sexual life agreed with the assertions he had made in the *Three Essays.* There Freud had made a distinction between two phases of childhood masturbation. An initial phase in early infancy—before a genital zone had acquired dominance—seemed "to disappear after a short time"; a second phase began usually during the fourth year: "the sexual excitation of early infancy" returned and again sought satisfaction in masturbation.[90] Freud's picture of Hans exhibited the features of the second phase: the penis as dominant erotogenic zone and as the locus of masturbation. "He had been," Freud wrote, "in a state of intensified sexual excitement, the object of which was his mother . . . and he found . . . [a] channel of discharge for it by masturbating every evening and in that way obtaining gratification."[91]

Freud's description also delineated "components" of the boy's sexuality. He had initially arrived at the notion of component instincts from a discussion of perversions. Sadism he regarded as "the most common and the most significant. . . . The sexuality of most male human beings" contained "an element of *aggressiveness*—a desire to subjugate." In normal sexuality sadism was only one among many components, whereas in perversion sadism had "become independent and exaggerated" and had "usurped the leading position."[92]

With children sadism expressed itself in both deed and fantasy. Between the time Freud began to receive reports about Hans and when he actually wrote up the case, he published a paper drawing largely on the boy's material, a paper about his fantasies and those of his peers entitled "On the Sexual Theories of Children." Among such theories figured one which Freud called a *"sadistic view of coition"*—a child's view of parental intercourse in part influenced by "obscure memories" of what he had witnessed "while he was still in his first years and was sharing his parents' bedroom." (Hans slept there until he was four and a half years old.)

> They see it [intercourse] as something that the stronger participant is forcibly inflicting on the weaker, and they (especially boys) compare it to the romping familiar to them from their childish experience—romping which, incidentally, is not without a dash of sexual excitation. . . . They have interpreted the act of love as an act of violence.[93]

In the subsequent "Analysis of a Phobia" Freud drew attention to fantasies in which Hans's sadism appeared undisguised. (It was *"suppressed sadism"*: the boy "was not by any means a bad character; he was not even one of those children" who gave "free play" to a "propensity towards cruelty and violence.")[94] Near the end of the analysis, when Hans enjoyed discoursing freely on horses, he told his father about things he would like to do to them. He started with teasing and how that might be accomplished; he went on to whipping. The father reported the conversation:

> *Hans:* "Once I really did it. Once I had the whip, and whipped the horse, and it fell down and made a row with its feet."
> *I:* "Who let you? Had the coachman left the horse standing?"
> *Hans:* "It was just a horse from the stables."
> *I:* "Was there no one in the stables?"

> *Hans:* "Oh yes, Loisl." (The coachman.)
> *I:* "Did he let you?"
> *Hans:* "I talked nicely to him, and he said I might do it."
> *I:* "What did you say to him?"
> *Hans:* "Could I take the horse and whip it and shout at it. And he said 'Yes'."
> *I:* "Did you whip it a lot?"
> *Hans: "What I've told you isn't true in the least."*
> *I:* "You never took a horse out of the stables?"
> *Hans:* "Oh no."
> *I:* "But you wanted to."
> *Hans:* "Oh yes, wanted. I've thought it to myself."

He also thought to himself about beating his mother:

> *Hans:* "I should just like to beat her."
> *I:* "When did you ever see any one beating their Mummy?"
> *Hans:* "I've never seen any one do it, never in all my life."
> *I:* "And yet you'd just like to do it. How would you like to set about it?"
> *Hans:* "With a carpet-beater."[95]

When Freud came to summarize the case material and to add a theoretical gloss, he gave prominence to the boy's aggressive inclinations. At this point he was on the verge of providing a supplementary (or alternative) explanation for Hans's fear of his father. According to the explanation he had offered the boy himself, because Hans loved his mother and nourished hostile impulses against his father, he thought the father would in turn be angry, and an angry, vengeful father provoked fear in Hans. According to the second explanation the boy might well have projected his own hostile impulses into the external world. As early as 1895 Freud had speculated that in paranoia (considered as one of the neuropsychoses of defense) the offending or incompatible idea was warded off "by projecting its substance into the external world."[96] Perhaps Hans had projected his hostile impulses onto the parent of whom he was now afraid. When in *Inhibitions, Symptoms and Anxiety* (1926) Freud reviewed the case, he concluded: "Instead of aggressiveness on the part of the subject towards his father, there appeared aggressiveness . . . on the part of his father towards the subject."[97]

Impulses, fantasies—and now an object—were all soldered together.

They joined at the "heart of the case" of Little Hans and suggested to Freud a "nuclear complex in neuroses."[98]

.   .   .

On October 1, 1907, a twenty-nine-year-old man, university educated, who for years had been afflicted with obsessional ideas, showed up in Freud's consulting room. He mentioned, as an example, a compulsion to cut his throat with a straight razor. Just when "he was in the middle of a very hard piece of work the idea had occurred to him: 'If you received a command to take your examination this term at the first possible opportunity, you might manage to obey it. But if you were commanded to cut your throat . . ., what then?' He had at once become aware that this command had already been given, and was hurrying to the cupboard to fetch his razor."[99] Years of his life, he complained on first meeting Freud, had been wasted fighting against such compulsions, commands, and prohibitions. Years also, Freud may have thought, had been wasted as his prospective patient tried the various treatments generally prescribed for ailments like his.[100] Yet it was not these longstanding torments that had brought the young man to Freud.

During his second regular analytic session the young man recounted, in a disjointed fashion, what had precipitated his current crisis. The preceding August, while doing his stint as an Austrian reserve officer, he had lost his pince-nez and had wired his optician in Vienna for a replacement. Having sent the telegram, he fell into conversation with a Czech captain who told him of a terrible punishment practiced in the East. At this point the young man "broke off, got up from the sofa," and begged Freud "to spare him the recital of the details." Freud refused; he could not grant a request that violated what had become the fundamental injunction of psychoanalysis: say it aloud.[101]

> I went on to say that I would do all that I could, nevertheless, to guess the full meaning of any hints he gave me. Was he perhaps thinking of impalement?—"No, not that; . . . the criminal was tied up . . ."—he expressed himself so indistinctly that I could not immediately guess in what position—". . . a pot was turned upside down on his buttocks . . . some *rats* were put into it . . . and they . . ."—he had again got up, and was showing every sign of horror . . .—". . . *bored their way in* . . ."—

"Into his anus," I helped him out. . . . He proceeded with the greatest difficulty: "At that moment the idea flashed through my mind *that this was happening to a person who was very dear to me.*"[102]

The rat punishment, so it had dawned on him, would be visited not only upon a lady he dearly loved, but upon his father as well. (Here Freud dryly noted that "as his father had died many years previously," fear for him was even "more nonsensical" than fear for his lady.)[103] That evening, when the Czech captain had handed the young man his pince-nez, which in the meantime had arrived, and had told him to reimburse Lieutenant David, a "sanction" had taken shape in his mind: "do not repay the money lest the fantasy become real." Then, in a manner he found familiar, a countercommand had come to him: "you must return" the sum in question to Lieutenant David.[104] He had spent the rest of the day and the next trying to obey the second command. (An official at the post office, he soon discovered, not the lieutenant, had advanced the money for the pince-nez; nonetheless he had not wavered in his determination to put the small sum into David's hands.) And he spent the rest of that session and the next trying to narrate his tortured and tortuous efforts to repay the wrong person.

After the patient, who soon earned the sobriquet Rat Man, had been in treatment less than a month, Freud reported on its initial phase to the Wednesday Psychological Society. From time to time over the next half year he provided additional information, giving a brief account of his understanding of one obsession or another.[105] The following April, as he was preparing for the first International Psychoanalytic Congress, to be held at Salzburg, he again exploited material provided by the analysis of this patient. His original aim had been to describe a completed case, one that could "be viewed as a whole." But he had no such case at hand. (He had to abandon "the idea of the five-year-old boy because his neurosis, though resolving itself splendidly," hadn't "kept the deadline.")[106] Instead he decided to present what he regarded as a mere "potpourri of particular observations and general remarks on a case of obsessional neurosis."[107] According to Ernest Jones that presentation kept his audience enthralled.

He [Freud] sat at the end of a long table along the sides of which we were all gathered and spoke in his usual low but distinct conversational tone. He began at . . . eight in the morning and we listened with rapt attention. At eleven he broke off, suggesting we had had enough. But we were so absorbed that we insisted on his continuing, which he did until nearly one o'clock.[108]

Freud never did describe the completed case; nor did he manage to offer a view of it as a whole. In the early summer of 1909, having been seized by an impulse to write about "the Salzburg rat man," he lamented "how bungled" a reproduction of one of the "great art works of psychic nature" his paper was turning out to be.[109] In the end he provided his readers only "some fragmentary extracts" drawn from "notes made on the evening of the day of treatment"—process notes which survive and which supplement the published account.[110] (And in comparison with his other case histories, this one has generally been judged "chaotic and un-story-like.")[111] Even Freud's remarks on obsessional neurosis remained something of a potpourri. Before putting pen to paper he had expressed the hope of throwing a "full light on certain aspects" of that "truly complicated phenomenon";[112] by the time he finished he had to be content with "some disconnected statements of an aphoristic character."[113]

Among the Rat Man's own disconnected statements what stood out was a conflict between his love for his father and his love for his lady. This conflict Freud considered a "simplification."[114] It corresponded to "the normal vacillation between male and female" that characterized "every man's choice of a love object"; it corresponded to the "time-honoured question" asked of a child: "Which do you love most, Daddy or Mummy?" Usually the answer little by little lost its either/or quality. Among Freud's disconnected statements what stood out were his remarks on the "*chronic* co-existence of love and hatred, both directed towards the same person and both of the highest degree of intensity"; his patient had been "unmistakably victim to a conflict between love and hatred, in regard . . . to his lady and to his father" alike.[115] (Freud later picked up the term "ambivalence" from the Swiss psychiatrist Eugen Bleuler to denote such an "emotional configuration.")[116] Usually passionate love conquered hatred or was devoured by it. Not so in this particular case.

The Rat Man, who became known to posterity by this strange sobriquet rather than a pseudonym like Dora, Hans, or Paul (as he was actually called in the text), was in reality Dr. Ernst Lanzer.[117] (The doctorate was a law degree.) Born in Vienna in 1878, he was the fourth child and first son—three more children, including a brother, followed—born to middle-class Jewish parents, Heinrich and Rosa. Heinrich, who figured so prominently in his son's case history, was, according to Freud, "a most excellent man . . . distinguished by a hearty sense of humour and a kindly tolerance towards his fellow-men." That hearty sense of humor could verge on the vulgar. Before his marriage he had served as a noncommissioned officer and had retained "a *penchant* for using downright language." Ernst, with "his over-refined attitude . . . was manifestly ashamed of his father's simple and soldierly nature." He was also afraid of his father's temper. The older man could be "hasty and violent." That haste and violence "occasionally brought down the most severe castigation upon the children." Still when Ernst grew up, he lived with his father "like the best of friends." And when he died, eight years before Ernst came to Freud, his son had been unable to accept the fact of his death.

> It had constantly happened to him that, when he heard a good joke, he would say to himself: "I must tell Father that." His imagination, too, had been occupied with his father, so that often, when there was a knock at the door, he would think: "Here comes Father," and when he walked into a room he would expect to find his father in it. And although he had never forgotten that his father was dead, the prospect of seeing a ghostly apparition of this kind had had no terrors for him; on the contrary, he had greatly desired it.[118]

In his published account Freud said practically nothing about Ernst's mother. Yet she was the one doling out the fees for her son's analytic treatment, a treatment which, after less than a year, made it possible for him to face "life with courage and ability."[119] (He was killed a few years later, during the First World War.)

Both Ernst and Freud approached their work together with quite definite expectations. Ernst knew something about Freud's theories, enough to assume that his physician would inquire about his sexual life, and at the very first interview the patient proceeded, without any prompting, to tell him that that life had been "stunted": masturbation played "a small part in it"; as for intercourse, he had first experienced it at the age of twenty-six, and thereafter "only at irregular intervals."

Part way into his first analytic session, the following day, he returned to this subject—"without any apparent transition":

> "My sexual life began very early. I can remember a scene during my fourth or fifth year. . . . We had a very pretty young governess. . . . One evening she was lying on the sofa lightly dressed, and reading. I was lying beside her, and begged her to let me creep under her skirt. She told me I might, so long as I said nothing to any one about it. She had very little on, and I fingered her genitals and the lower part of her body, which struck me as very queer. After this I was left with a burning and tormenting curiosity to see the female body. . . .
>
> There were certain people, girls, who pleased me very much, and I had a very strong wish *to see them naked*. But in wishing this I had an *uncanny feeling, as though something might happen if I thought such things, and as though I must do all sorts of things to prevent it.*"
>
> (In reply to a question he gave an example of these fears: "For instance, *that my father might die.*")

Picking up again the theme of his sexual life, Ernst began the sixth session by recounting, with some urgency, an event of his youth:

> When he was twelve years old he had been in love with a little girl, the sister of a friend. . . . But she had not shown him as much affection as he had desired. And thereupon the idea had come to him that she would be kind to him if some misfortune were to befall him; and as an instance of such a misfortune his father's death had forced itself upon his mind. . . . He then proceeded to tell me that a precisely similar thought had flashed through his mind a second time, six months before his father's death. At that time he had already been in love with his lady, but financial obstacles made it impossible to think of an alliance with her. The idea had then occurred to him that *his father's death might make him rich enough to marry her*. . . . The same idea, though in a much milder form, had come to him for a third time, on the day before his father's death. He had then thought: "Now I may be going to lose what I love most;" and then had come the contradiction: "No, there is someone else whose loss would be even more painful to you." These thoughts surprised him very much, for he was quite certain that his father's death could never have been an object of his desire but only of his fear.[120]

At this point Freud began to give some hint of his own quite definite expectations. Initially he had been prepared to find hostility toward the father and was convinced, as he told Ernst, that behind fear of his father's dying lay a death-wish that had been energetically repudiated; and indeed the very intensity of Ernst's love for his father signaled a repressed (and equally intense) hatred. In addition Freud assumed that the hatred must have a source and that that source had something to do with *"sensual desires."*[121] "Hatred for the father as strong as in this case," Freud reported to the members of the Wednesday Psychological Society, could "arise only if the father" had "disturbed the child in his sexuality."[122]

In a session during which Ernst returned to the subject of his sexual life, Freud offered a possible "construction" of what had happened. His patient had told of "curiosity" about masturbation coming "over him in his twenty-first year, *shortly after his father's death.*" He had told of the shame he had felt "each time he gave way to this kind of gratification" and of the vow he had made to foreswear such activities. It had been a self-imposed prohibition that he had not abided by. He had told of the occasions on which he had violated it, and Freud "could not help pointing out that these . . . occasions had something in common—a prohibition, and the defiance of a command." Prompted by this material, Freud suggested that when Ernst "was a child of under six" he had been "soundly castigated by his father" for masturbation; the masturbation had come to an end, but the punishment "had left behind . . . an ineradicable grudge against his father and had established him for all time in his role of an interferer with the patient's sexual enjoyment."[123] Once again, like an archeologist, Freud was trying to "bring to the light of day after their long burial the priceless . . . relics of antiquity."[124]

Ernst responded to this construction by reporting a childhood scene which he himself did not recall, but which had been repeatedly described to him by his mother. "The tale was as follows."

> When he was very small . . . he had done something naughty, for which his father had given him a beating. The little boy had flown into a terrible rage and had hurled abuse at his father even while he was under his blows. But as he knew no bad language, he had called him by all the names of common objects that he could think of, and had screamed: "You lamp! You towel! You plate!" and so on. His father, shaken by such an outburst of elemental fury, had stopped beating him, and had declared: "The child will be either a great man or a great criminal!" . . . His father, he said,

never beat him again; and he also attributed to this experience . . . the change which came over his own character. From that time forward he was a coward—out of fear of the violence of his own rage.[125]

Was this the relic Freud had hoped to find? Almost, but not quite. When Ernst checked with his mother, she confirmed the story, but added that he had been punished for biting someone, not for masturbating. The mother's testimony alone, Freud argued in a long footnote, was not, however, reason enough to abandon his insistence on childhood sexuality.

The hostility toward the father, or rather ambivalence—the love was assumed—Freud insisted on tracing back to childhood; the hostility or ambivalence toward the lady Ernst loved had everything of today about it. (Only in the long footnote defending his claims about childhood sexuality did Freud refer to Ernst's "desires for his mother." In the text itself he neglected entirely the connection between mother and lady.)[126] As to the source of those feelings, Freud thought the answer obvious: the lady had twice rejected Ernst's proposals of marriage. The second rejection had prompted a number of obsessional activities, among them his removing a stone from the road over which her carriage would shortly pass, lest the carriage "come to grief" against it, and then twenty minutes later putting it back again.[127] (They married in 1910.)

A year later Freud set the asymmetry right. In a paper entitled "A Special Type of Choice of Object Made by Men," he described an "object-choice derived from the infantile fixation . . . on the mother." As a consequence of that fixation "maternal characteristics" remained "stamped" on later love objects, all of whom were "easily recognizable" as "mother-surrogates." Two characteristics—or "preconditions for loving"—stood out: first, the "woman should not be unattached" or there "should be an injured third party"; second, she "should be like a prostitute." That the first condition was backward-looking seemed readily apparent: "It is at once clear that for the child who is growing up in the family circle the fact of the mother belonging to the father becomes an inseparable part of the mother's essence, and . . . the injured third party is none other than the father himself." The second condition could also be traced back to childhood, to the time when the boy began to have sexual impulses toward his mother (seeking relief in masturbation) and began to hate his father as a rival, that is to say, when he came "under the dominance of the Oedipus complex." It was a time when the boy blamed "his mother for having granted the favour of sexual intercourse not to himself but to his father," and he regarded it as "an act of unfaithfulness."[128] In short, he regarded his mother as no better than a whore. Here Freud seemed to be drawing on material from Ernst's case, from material contained in the process notes, not the text. When his lady had rejected his marriage proposal a second time, "his fury against her had been tremendous," and he remembered thinking that she was a whore. "Whore," Freud commented parenthetically, pointed to "a comparison with his mother."[129]

It was in this paper on object-choice that Freud coined the famous name by which the "nuclear complex of the neuroses" came to be known.[130] The Oedipus complex—choosing mother (or her surrogate) over father (the simplification Ernst recognized as the choice between lady and father)—represented a streamlining of relationships with two objects toward whom the child felt both love and hate.

.   .   .

> The uniformity . . . of the sexual life of children . . . will easily account for the constant sameness which as a rule characterizes the phantasies that are constructed around the period of childhood, irrespective of how greatly or how little real experiences have contributed towards them.[131]

Thanks to such sexually saturated fantasies, Freud continued, the child fashioned the oedipal father—and, he might have added, the oedipal mother as well. What role did history, that is, the child's actual experiences, play in such fashioning? So long as Freud thought of fantasy as distorted memory, he persevered in his attempt to uncover the historical past. And he never stopped thinking of fantasy in that way. Yet alongside this notion, or entwined with it, another conceptual strand became increasingly prominent: fantasy soldered to impulse, or fantasy as a (disguised) expression of impulse. Fantasies, so construed, dampened Freud's ardor for determining whether childhood experiences reported in analysis should be reckoned reality or fantasy.[132]

An Altered Ego

At the climax of his illness, under the influence of visions which were "partly of a terrifying character, but partly too, of an indescribable grandeur," Schreber became convinced of the imminence of a great catastrophe, of the end of the world. Voices told him that the work of the past 14,000 years had now come to nothing, and that the earth's allotted span was only 212 years more; and during the last part of his stay in . . . [the] clinic he believed that that period had already elapsed. He himself was "the only real man left alive," and the few human shapes that he saw—the doctor, the attendants, the other patients—he explained as being "miracled up, cursorily improvised men." Years afterwards, when Dr. Schreber . . . returned to human society, . . . he could not bring himself to doubt that during his illness the world had come to an end and that, in spite of everything, the one that he now saw before him was a different one.[133]

Freud seized on the image of "world-catastrophe." It represented, he argued, the "projection" of an "internal catastrophe": Schreber had detached his libido from external objects, that is, he had withdrawn his love "from people in his environment," and this detachment or withdrawal had destroyed his world. His *"delusional formation"* of becoming a woman represented *"an attempt at recovery, a process of reconstruction"*: he had begun to build anew so that he could at least live in a world once more.[134]

Detaching libido might be catastrophic—or it might not. Freud did not regard such detachment as peculiar to paranoia: in "normal mental life" one withdrew love from people "without falling ill"; a "normal person" would "at once begin looking about for a substitute for the lost attachment." The crucial point was what happened to the liberated or detached libido in the meantime. In the normal person it would simply be "kept in suspension"; in the person suffering from paranoia it would be "put to a special use": it would be "attached to the ego" and be exploited for the ego's "aggrandizement."[135]

Here Freud took another step, or rather claimed that Schreber had taken one: in detaching his libido, Freud argued, he had taken a step backward, to narcissism. (Regression to narcissism, Freud next maintained, was characteristic of paranoia.)[136] In the 1905 edition of the *Three Essays* stages in the development of object love had not been specified. Freud had described auto-erotism as infantile sexuality no longer linked to "the taking of nourishment" and no longer requiring an external object. He had also discussed finding, or refinding, an object, a process not completed until puberty. During the intervening years the child loved those taking care of him with what Freud described as "damped-down libido."[137] In writing about Schreber, he designated auto-erotism and object-love as stages and interpolated narcissism between them.

What did this new stage signify? The chief novelty lay in the introduction of the ego as object: the ego itself could be the "person's only sexual object."[138] Even more than in the case of the sequence oral, anal, and phallic, the reader was well advised not to construe this progression too rigidly. Narcissism and object-love did not overlap; rather they seesawed back and forth. And in that seesawing, Freud subsequently suggested, "the shadow" of an object soldered together with sexually saturated fantasy "fell upon the ego."[139]

.   .   .

> Being enamoured of oneself (of one's own genitals) is an indispensable stage of development. . . . In general, man has two primary sexual objects, and his future existence depends on which of these objects he remains fixated on. These two sexual objects are for every man the woman (the mother, nurse, etc.) and his own person; and it follows from this that [the question] is to become free from both and not to linger too long with either.[140]

The case presented in November 1909 to the Vienna Psychoanalytic Society, which provoked Freud's intervention, was one of "multiform perversion," and the "perversion" that elicited the most discussion was homosexuality. On December 1, 1909, Freud himself delivered a paper which served to flesh out the comments he had made a month earlier. Its theoretical focus was on latent homosexuality; its clinical focus was on Leonardo da Vinci.

In tackling a historical figure Freud once again sounded the note of a conquistador. This time he had comrades-in-arms whom he exhorted to "conquer the whole field of mythology" and to "take hold of biography." His own chosen battle plan was to attack "the riddle" of Leonardo. It would be, he recognized, a risky undertaking. "The material concerning L.," he wrote one of his comrades, was "so sparse" that he despaired of "demonstrating . . . intelligibly" his "conviction" about it.[141] When in 1910 he actually published his study, he sounded a modest note: he took pains to make clear that conquest in "the field of biography" was beyond his reach. The "fragmentary nature" of the information relating to Leonardo, he noted, meant that in this case a psychoanalytic biography could not "provide any certain results." But the fault lay with himself alone; he bore the responsibility for "having forced psycho-analysis to pronounce an expert opinion on the basis of such insufficient material."[142] This was no reason to call psychoanalysis itself into question.

Freud's interest in Leonardo was longstanding. In 1898, at a time when Fliess was investigating left-handedness, Freud mentioned the Renaissance figure as "perhaps the most famous left-handed person." He also mentioned that "no love affair of his" was "known."[143] In 1907, when asked to name ten good books, Freud included Dmitry Merezhkovsky's *Leonardo da Vinci*.[144] From the use he made of that historical romance in his own study, one can infer that it was the vivid account this "psychological novelist" gave of Leonardo's love life that earned Freud's esteem. The artist may never have "embraced a woman in passion," but "he surrounded himself with handsome boys and youths whom he took as pupils"—without those "affectionate relations" extending to "sexual activity."[145] Thus when in 1909 Freud came across Leonardo's "image and likeness (without his genius) in a neurotic," this "sexually inactive or homosexual" patient's case prompted him to wrestle with the riddle of Leonardo and in so doing make graphic his understanding of latent homosexuality.[146]

The whole study hinged on interpreting a single childhood memory. Leonardo had inserted it in one of his scientific notebooks, and it was the only bit of information about his childhood, as far as Freud knew, that he had so included. It was a recollection of the "strangest sort"— strange alike in content and in the age to which it had been assigned. "I recall as one of my earliest memories that while I was in my cradle a vulture came down to me, and opened my mouth with its tail, and struck me many times with its tail against my lips."[147] (The German translation from which Freud was working had mistaken a kite for a vulture. Hence his pursuit of the vulture in Egyptian mythology turned out to be a wild goose chase.)

Did this recollection accurately capture a historical event? Freud had no difficulty answering in the negative. In the case of his own memory of the green meadow with yellow flowers, he had been tempted to conclude that it had been constructed like a work of fiction. In the case of Leonardo, given the fabulous nature of the recollection, the temptation was overwhelming: it had been manufactured, Freud argued, like a work of history itself, in particular the "history of a nation's earliest days, . . . compiled later and for tendentious reasons." Did Leonardo's recollection, then, contain no historical truth? Again Freud answered in the negative. He was confident that crucial elements of the artist's childhood could be extracted from what was clearly a "phantasy from a later period."[148]

Freud concentrated on the vulture's tail—an obvious phallus. Both mythology and children's sexual theories, he claimed, demonstrated that the "human imagination" did not "boggle at endowing a figure," which was "intended to embody the essence of the mother, with the mark of male potency." And its appearance in Leonardo's recollection allowed Freud to extract from it a species of historical truth: he had been suckled by a mother whom he fantasized as phallic. (It was well known that Leonardo had been born out of wedlock; it was also known that by the age of five he was resident in the household of his father and stepmother.) Freud now argued that Leonardo had spent the intervening years "with his poor, forsaken, real mother," and that he had "had time to feel the absence of his father." The vulture's tail also pointed "to the idea of an act of *fellatio*" and thus resembled "certain dreams and phantasies found in women or passive homosexuals." From it Freud proceeded to extract another species of historical truth:

> In words which only too plainly recall a description of a sexual act ("and struck me many times with its tail against my lips"), Leonardo stresses the intensity of the erotic relations between mother and child. From this linking of his mother's (the vulture's) activity with the prominence of the mouth zone it is not difficult to guess that a second memory is contained in the phantasy. This may be translated: "My mother pressed innumerable passionate kisses on my mouth." The phantasy is compounded from the memory of being suckled and being kissed by his mother.[149]

Could there be something in Leonardo's life work that bore witness to what Freud had unearthed "as the strongest impression of his childhood?" Mona Lisa del Giocondo's smile was Freud's answer. It had awakened in the adult painter "the memory of the mother of earliest childhood." The "unchanging smile, on long, curved lips" was blissful; it was sinister as well. Following the lead of art critics, Freud saw in it two distinct elements—precisely the ones which dominated "the erotic life of women; . . . the most devoted tenderness and a sensuality that is ruthlessly demanding—consuming men as if they were alien beings." And so it had been, he surmised, with Leonardo's mother:

> In her love for her child the poor forsaken mother had to give vent to all her memories of the caresses she had enjoyed as well as her longing for new ones; and she was forced to do so not only to compensate herself for having no husband, but also to compensate her child for having no father to fondle him. So, like all unsatisfied mothers, she took her little son in place of her husband, and by the too early maturing of his erotism robbed him of a part of his masculinity.[150]

Could Leonardo's "later manifest, if ideal, homosexuality" be made to fit Freud's surmise? Instead of finding an erotic substitute for his mother, Leonardo put himself in her place; he loved boys the way his mother had "loved *him* when he was a child." His pupils, selected not for their talent but for their beauty, "he treated . . . with kindness and consideration, looked after them, and when they were ill nursed them himself, . . . just as his . . . mother might have tended him." In so doing he was taking "his own person as a model" for the "new objects of his love": the boys whom he now loved were surrogate "figures and revivals of himself in childhood."[151] What he was searching for was his "own childhood ego."[152] Identification with his mother and choosing himself as love object went hand in hand.[153]

Like Narcissus, Leonardo lingered too long over his reflection. He also lingered too long over his mother. (A man, Freud claimed, who became homosexual the way Leonardo had, remained "unconsciously fixated to the mnemic image of his mother.")[154] In this case a smile, not a shadow, had fallen upon the ego.

.   .   .

When in February 1910 Sergei Pankejeff first encountered Freud, the twenty-three-year-old Russian, scion of an enormously wealthy landed family, was suffering from a serious disorder—how to label it still remains a matter of dispute. Freud himself offered neither a description of the presenting symptoms nor an exact diagnosis; he merely stated that his new patient was "entirely incapacitated and completely dependent upon other people."[155] He had in fact arrived in Vienna accompanied by a medical student and a psychiatrist from Odessa, who knew something of psychoanalysis and hence sought out Freud's help for his patient. These two attendants remained on hand until late in the year, by which time Sergei was obliged or able to manage minimally on his own.

His family included a number of seriously disturbed individuals, whose illnesses impinged on Sergei's childhood. He remembered and reported to Freud that in his earliest years he and his father had enjoyed a close and affectionate tie; the little boy had been proud of the older man and had frequently declared that "he would like to be a gentleman like him." The two had subsequently become estranged, and Sergei's "maturer years were marked by a very unsatisfactory relation to his father, who, after repeated attacks of depression, was no longer able to conceal the pathological features of his character."[156] The ill-health of Sergei's mother had become manifest much sooner, in abdominal pains and hemorrhages and also in hypochondria, all of which had prevented her from having much to do with either her daughter or her son. Her health improved as time went on, and she lived to the age of eighty-seven. The daughter, Anna—two and a half years older than her brother—was gifted and tempestuous, and her father's favorite. Sergei himself described her as behaving "less like a little girl than like a naughty boy," and indeed he was often told as a child that he ought to have been the girl and Anna the boy.[157] Among her many talents was a knack for tormenting her brother, for exploiting his fears and then delighting in his expression of terror. In this Dostoyevskian household only his beloved Nanya, a devout peasant, seemed truly attached to him.

According to Freud, his patient had "broken down in his eighteenth year after a gonorrhoeal infection."[158] Between then and his consultation with Freud, Sergei's sister committed suicide, and his father died, possibly also a suicide. During those same years he sampled the best of European psychiatry and its sanatoria. He visited the leading neurologist in St. Petersburg, who labeled him a neurasthenic and recommended hypnosis. The treatment worked wonders—for one whole day. He was escorted to Munich to be examined by the preeminent German psychiatrist Emil Kraepelin, who had earned his renown by bringing order into psychiatric nosology. (Kraepelin had periodically treated Sergei's father and judged that both father and son were manic-depressive.) He recommended an extended stay in a sanatorium. There Sergei fell in love with a nurse named Therese and courted her compulsively. Back and forth he went, to his inamorata and away from her, from Germany to Russia and from Russia to Germany. Eventually his psychiatric sampling took him to Berlin and to Theodor Ziehen, then chief of the Charité Hospital. Again the psychiatrist recommended an extended stay in a sanatorium, and again Sergei decamped, owing to the vicissitudes of his love life. When he showed up in Freud's consulting room, both his mental and his amorous states had something protean about them.

Sergei not only showed up in Freud's consulting room—he remained until June 1914. In contrast to relatives and psychiatrists alike, who had uniformly advised him to sever his tie to Therese, Freud offered no such advice. When Sergei told his new therapist of the turbulent courtship and asked whether he should continue the pursuit, Freud replied in the affirmative "but with the condition that this would take place only after several months of analysis." According to Sergei, Freud regarded his attachment as "the breakthrough to the woman," and "under certain circumstances" a breakthrough of this sort "could be considered the neurotic's greatest achievement, a sign of his will to live, an active attempt to recover."[159] Freud's own clinical focus fastened on his patient's latent homosexuality. (In contrast to Leonardo, who had suffered from the absence of a strong father in childhood, Sergei had suffered from a paternal presence.) At the beginning of treatment, few of his patient's "psychical trends," Freud wrote, had been "concentrated in his heterosexual object-choice," and "his homosexual attitude . . . persisted in him as an unconscious force with . . . very great intensity." In these circumstances, that is, in light of what Freud regarded as his patient's "inhibited sexual development," he was prepared to sanction Sergei's "fight for the object of his masculine desires."[160]

That fight proved to be lifelong. A year into the analysis, Freud at last consented to Sergei's reunion with Therese. In accordance, however, with his rule that a patient "promise not to take any important decisions affecting his life during . . . treatment,"[161] marriage was postponed until after termination—which coincided with the assassination of the Archduke Franz Ferdinand. Stormy world-historical events ensued. In memoirs written toward the end of his life Sergei did not reveal whether, on the personal level, further storms had followed an unsettled and unsettling courtship. In interviews granted to an Austrian journalist a couple of years before his death in 1979, he made good his omission:

> I wanted Therese, Therese excited me sexually. . . . But then what? I went away, I came back to her and what did I find? She was broken in health, emaciated like a skeleton. . . .
> I forced myself. . . . You see, and that was the bad thing now, this is a secret, what I am telling you, now I looked for the sexual in other women. I loved her, and with other women it was the sexual thing. But that had nothing to do with her suicide. Hitler had something to do with her suicide.[162]

Therese killed herself in 1938, shortly after German troops marched into Vienna, and shortly before Freud himself emigrated.

Sergei's involvement with psychoanalysis also proved to be lifelong. It did not end in 1914; it did not end in 1938. In his words, he became "a showpiece of psychoanalysis,"[163] and until his death psychoanalysts continued to give him therapeutic and even financial support. He had returned to Vienna in 1919 for further work with Freud, because, he wrote, "there was still a small residue of unanalyzed material."[164] That reanalysis lasted until the spring of the following year. (There was nothing left of his vast fortune, but he managed to find employment as a minor functionary in an insurance company in Vienna and held that job for almost thirty years.) In 1926 paranoid delusions drove him back into analysis, this time with Ruth Mack Brunswick, who was herself in analysis with Freud. Sergei's treatment lasted roughly five months. Two years later he resumed analysis with Mack Brunswick, and it continued intermittently for several more years. In 1938, after Therese's suicide, a distraught Sergei pursued his therapist to Paris and London for a few weeks of treatment. After the Second World War he was in irregular contact with Muriel Gardiner and from the mid-1950s on in regular contact with Kurt Eissler, who spent a number of weeks each summer in Vienna. Together Eissler and Sergei engaged in daily analytically oriented conversations. From this history of treatment it is easy to conclude that analysis had failed to rehabilitate the patient; instead it had become a new form of dependency. How Sergei would have fared without psychoanalysis, one has no way of judging.

His lifelong involvement did not necessarily make him the showpiece of analysis; the fact that Freud published his case constituted a much more significant contribution. Sergei had urged his analyst to write up a "complete history of his illness." Freud had demurred: such a history was "technically impracticable and socially impermissible." Instead he chose to concentrate on "a severe neurotic disturbance" that had dominated Sergei's "earlier years": it had begun "immediately before his fourth birthday as an anxiety-hysteria (in the shape of an animal phobia), then changed into an obsessional neurosis . . . and lasted with offshoots . . . into his tenth year." To justify dealing "with an infantile neurosis . . . not while it actually existed but only fifteen years after its termination," Freud advanced an argument that smacked of special pleading—all the more so in view of what and when he had written about Little Hans:

> An analysis which is conducted upon a neurotic child itself must, as a matter of course, appear to be more trustworthy, but it cannot be very rich in material; too many words and thoughts have to be lent to the child, and even so the deepest strata may turn out to be impenetrable to consciousness. An analysis of a childhood disorder through the medium of recollection in an intellectually mature adult is free from these limitations; but it necessitates our taking into account the distortion and refurbishing to which a person's own past is subjected when it is looked back upon from a later period. The first alternative perhaps gives the more convincing results; the second is by far the more instructive.[165]

Freud was intent on being instructive.

The position that he set out to defend was absolutely central: the etiological significance of childhood experience. The seduction hypothesis had ranked as a first and abortive attempt to find a causal role for such experience; the turn to sexuality figured as the beginning of a second effort; and the articulation of the Oedipus complex, its designation as the "nuclear complex of the neuroses," represented the crucial next step. Freud then clinched the argument by asserting that "every neurosis in an adult is built upon a neurosis which has occurred in his childhood but has not invariably been severe enough to strike the eye and be recognized as such."[166] No wonder that he regarded as betrayal and attack the defection of Carl Gustav Jung—especially the Swiss psychiatrist's denial of the neuroses' childhood origin. In 1914, with this defection (as well as that of Alfred Adler) in mind, he wrote up his incomplete account of Sergei's case under the title "From the History of an Infantile Neurosis"; it was not actually published until 1918.

Pride of place in Freud's account belonged to a dream, the most famous dream dreamt by a patient in psychoanalytic literature. Its interpretation led to unraveling the complexities of Sergei's infantile sexuality; at the same time, Freud argued, the dream itself marked a crucial point in that sexual history, a point at which Sergei remained fixed—transfixed with terror that a wolf would gobble him up. Here is the dream Sergei dreamt as a small child and reported to Freud at an "early stage of the analysis" almost two decades later:

> *I dreamt that it was night and that I was lying in my bed. . . . Suddenly the window opened of its own accord, and I was terrified to see that some white wolves were sitting on the big walnut tree in front of the window. There were six or seven of them. The wolves were quite white, and looked more like foxes or sheep-dogs, for they had big tails like foxes and they had their ears pricked like dogs when they pay attention to something. . . . I screamed.*[167]

The dream may have turned up early in the analysis; it was, however, only during the last months of treatment "that it became possible to understand it completely." How had Freud arrived at that under-standing? He shied away from a meticulous reckoning; he offered no technical display of dream interpretation; he relegated his attempt at a "comprehensive account of the relation between the manifest content of the dream and the latent dream-thoughts" to a long footnote. All the same "the lasting sense of reality" which the dream had left behind convinced Freud that "some part of the latent material" related to an event which had actually taken place and had not been "merely imagined."[168] Like an archeologist, he had resolved to uncover the histori-cal past that in this instance lay beneath a dream. (Before publishing his account, he interpolated that whether what had emerged was an experience or a fantasy was not "a matter of great importance." And then he added: "Scenes of observing parental intercourse, of being seduced in childhood, and of being threatened with castration" were "unquestionably an inherited endowment, a phylogenetic heritage.")[169]

A "provisional" analysis, Freud wrote, had supplied him with grounds for a fragmentary reconstruction: a *"real occurrence"*—derived from "the lasting sense of reality"; *"dating from a very early period"*— based on Sergei's recollection (subsequently he associated the walnut tree to a Christmas tree—he had been born on Christmas—enabling Freud to fix the date of the dream as just before his fourth birthday); *"looking—immobility"*—from the manifest content (later Sergei himself interpreted the window opening of its own accord as meaning that his eyes suddenly opened, and that he, not the wolves, was attentively looking; Freud followed suit, suggesting that the wolves' immobility was also a reversal, and that they were actually engaged in "the most violent motion"); *sexual problems*—based on evidence of Sergei's childhood "sexual researches"; *"castration"*—from a fairy tale Sergei knew well at the time; *"his father"*—based on Freud's hunch that a "wolf may have been a father-surrogate"; *"something terrible"*—Sergei's own terror underwrote the last fragment.[170]

At this point in his exposition Freud abandoned his effort to trace the steps from the merely provisional and expressed the fear that his "reader's belief" would abandon him.

> What sprang into activity that night out of the chaos of the dreamer's unconscious memory-traces was the picture of copulation between his parents. . . . It gradually became possible to find satisfactory answers to all the questions that arose in connection with this scene. . . . Thus in the first place the child's age at the date of the observation was established as being about one and a half years. He was suffering at the time from malaria, an attack of which used to come on every day at a particular hour. . . . Probably for the very reason of this illness, he was in his parents' bedroom. . . . He had been sleeping in his cot . . . and woke up, perhaps because of his rising fever, in the afternoon. . . . It harmonizes with our assumption that it was a hot summer's day, if we suppose that his parents had retired, half undressed, for . . . [a] *siesta*. When he woke up, he witnessed a coitus *a tergo* [from behind], three times repeated; he was able to see his mother's genitals as well as his father's organ.[171]

How did parental intercourse come to be represented by six or seven wolves sitting in a tree? Material from a fairy tale Sergei had been told shortly before, Freud suggested, offered the necessary cover: its recent date and indifferent content meant that it was available as a node and point of entry for an intense unconscious wish. A tailor, so the story went, had been "at work in his room, when the window opened and a wolf leapt in." He caught the intruder by his tail and yanked it off. Some time later, walking in a forest, he saw a pack of wolves, the maimed one among them, coming toward him. To escape he scrambled up a tree. Intent on revenge, the maimed wolf organized an attack: he proposed that his pack-mates "should climb one upon another till the last one" reached the target. "He himself—he was a vigorous old fellow—would be the base of the pyramid." The tailor recognized the ringleader and called out: "'Catch the grey one by his tail!' The tailless wolf, terrified by the recollection, ran away, and all the others tumbled down." (In the dream the wolves came equipped with especially bushy tails, a disguise and reversal of taillessness.) What connected the "content of the primal scene to that of the wolf story"? Posture, Freud claimed, provided the associative bridge. It was the detail of the maimed wolf asking "the others *to climb upon him*" that evoked coitus *a tergo;* it thus became possible for the wolf story to represent parental intercourse and for "*several* wolves" to replace "*two* parents."[172]

Once Freud had drawn a primal scene replete with actors and action, he could bring to life his understanding of Sergei's sexuality. At the time of the dream, that is, at the age of four, the boy's most ardent wish, he argued, had been for sexual satisfaction from his father, not his mother, and it was this wish that had instigated the dream. In so doing it had revived a long-forgotten memory which graphically demonstrated "what sexual satisfaction from father was like." Instead of pleasure, however, the boy experienced terror—terror so great that he repressed "his over-powerful homosexuality." The result of "the dream was not so much the triumph of a masculine current, as a reaction against a feminine . . . one."[173]

What lay at the origin of Sergei's "over-powerful homosexuality"? Freud's account fell into two parts. In the first he pointed to the fact—and he regarded it as a fact not a fantasy—that when Sergei was roughly three and a half, at a time when his father was away from home, his sister, remembered in the family as a "forward and sensual

little thing," had "seduced him into sexual practices." The "seduction," Freud claimed, had given Sergei "the passive sexual aim of being
touched on the genitals." His patient recalled fantasies dating from this
period "of boys being chastised and beaten, and especially being
beaten on the penis," and they confirmed, in Freud's mind, the preva-
lence of such passive or masochistic tendencies. (He equated the two.)
The seduction, then, profoundly influenced Sergei's sexual aim; it did
not, however, determine what figured as the second part of Freud's
account: the choice of object. When his father returned, Sergei transferred to him "a passive attitude"—a stance he had first taken toward
his sister, then toward his Nanya, both of whom discouraged him in
one way or another. He now sought to have his beating fantasies
enacted. Through fits of naughtiness he tried "to force punishments
. . . out of his father"; he recalled how, during one of these fits, "he
had redoubled his screams as soon as his father" came near. His father,
alas, "did not beat him"; Sergei did not "obtain from him the masochistic sexual satisfaction he desired."[174]

What made him repress the desire for such satisfaction? The simple
answer was a threat of castration. But not any threatener would do.
When, after his sister had inducted Sergei into "sexual practices," he
had attempted to seduce his Nanya by playing with his penis in her
presence, and she had responded by making a "serious face" and
warning him that "children who did that . . . got a 'wound' in the
place," he had not been deterred. He still had "no belief" in castration
and had "no dread of it." The dream-induced activation of the primal
scene changed all that. Sergei now reacted "adequately" to the impression he had received at the age of one and a half: he now "saw with
his own eyes the wound of which his Nanya had spoken": "'If you
want to be sexually satisfied by Father,' we may perhaps represent him
as saying to himself, 'you must allow yourself to be castrated like
Mother; but I won't have that!'"[175] Sergei remained sufficiently enam-
oured of his own genitals to relinquish "his wish to be loved by his
father."[176]

Before the dream he had not believed in the reality of castration; he
also had had no fear of wolves. The dream changed that too. There
was a particular picture-book in which a wolf was portrayed, "standing
upright and striding along" and the sight of which made him "scream
like a lunatic" that the wolf would eat him up. (His sister took delight

in forcing him to look at the picture.) And the fear of the wolf/father did not disappear, even though the animal phobia gave way to an obsessional neurosis. It constituted the "strongest motive" for Sergei's "falling ill, and his ambivalent attitude towards every father-surrogate was the dominating feature of his life as well as of his behaviour during treatment."[177] Ambivalent because, like Leonardo, Sergei's love lingered on in the unconscious, intense and unchanging.

"This is the Wolf-Man."[178] Thus did Sergei identify himself over the telephone to the Austrian journalist/interviewer. Had the terrifying shadow of the wolf/father—and of the analyst whose case history had suggested the sobriquet—fallen on his ego?

.　　　.　　　.

> An object-choice, an attachment of the libido to a particular person, had at one time existed; then, owing to a real slight or disappointment coming from the loved person, the object-relationship was shattered. . . . But the free libido was not displaced on to another object; it was withdrawn into the ego. There . . . it . . . served to establish an *identification* of the ego with the abandoned object.[179]

In the case of Schreber, Freud had conceptualized the withdrawal of libido as a regression to narcissism. Three years later, in his 1914 paper "On Narcissism: An Introduction," he had argued that the objects from which libido had been detached were not replaced by other objects, not even in fantasy.[180] In 1915, however, when he wrote the lines quoted above, he reassessed what such a regression entailed—without rethinking the case of Schreber. The ego now identified with the abandoned object—its shadow fell on the ego, it was incorporated into the ego—and the ego itself was altered by this identification.

Both Leonardo and Sergei had relinquished an object—an object that had been soldered together with sexually saturated fantasy; both had remained unconsciously tied to the mnemic image of that object; in short, in both cases the shadow of the object had fallen on the ego. How had those egos been changed? Leonardo had been "robbed . . . of a part of his masculinity"; Sergei had been blocked on his way to it.[181] Once again anatomy and destiny had parted company.

CHAPTER FOUR

Modes of Conversation

> The confession is a ritual of discourse . . . that unfolds within a power relationship, for one does not confess without the presence (or virtual presence) of a partner who is not simply the interlocutor but the authority who requires the confession, prescribes and appreciates it, and intervenes in order to judge, punish, forgive, console, and reconcile; a ritual in which the truth is corroborated by the obstacles and resistances it has had to surmount in order to be formulated; and finally, a ritual in which the expression alone, independently of its external consequences, produces intrinsic modifications in the person who articulates it.

This ritual of discourse, Michel Foucault wrote, "spread its effects far and wide."[1] It spread to pedagogy, criminology, medicine, and the science of sexuality. That there might be a family resemblance among these enterprises and psychoanalysis should come as no surprise. What Foucault did was to borrow from psychoanalysis to provide an account of confessional technologies.[2]

How did Freud understand the analytic relationship? Simply to rehearse his explicit statements would be inadequate. Practice, not theory, was the crux of the matter. From the outset that practice was bound up with sexuality, and sexuality filled the analytic relationship with sound and fury. Initially—both as doctor and, paradoxically enough, as patient in his own "self-analysis"—Freud encountered this tempest and failed to master it. Eventually he succeeded in rethinking mastery itself and was then able to suggest how a "ritual of discourse" might produce "modifications" in the patient.

"New" or "Revised Editions"

> What really happened with Breuer's patient [Anna O.] I was able to guess later on, long after the break in our relations, when I suddenly remembered something Breuer had once told me in another context. . . . On the evening of the day when all her symptoms had been disposed of, he was summoned to the patient again, found her confused and writhing in abdominal cramps. Asked what was wrong with her, she replied: "Now Dr. B.'s child is coming!"
>
> At this moment he held in his hand the key . . . , but he let it drop. With all his great intellectual gifts there was nothing Faustian in his nature. Seized by conventional horror he took flight and abandoned the patient to a colleague.[3]

In the above letter to Stefan Zweig, written in 1932, Freud spelled out in detail what he had merely hinted at earlier in print.[4] To Ernest Jones he was equally explicit, and thanks to Jones this version, with embellishment, became orthodoxy in the history of psychoanalysis.

> It would seem that Breuer had developed . . . a strong [attachment] . . . to his interesting patient. At all events he was so engrossed that his wife became . . . jealous. She did not display this openly, but became unhappy and morose. It was a long time before Breuer, with his thoughts elsewhere, divined the meaning of her state of mind. It provoked a violent reaction in him, perhaps compounded of love and guilt, and he decided to bring the treatment to an end. He announced this to Anna O., who was by now much better, and bade her good-by. But that evening he was fetched back to find her in a greatly excited state, apparently as ill as ever. The patient, who according to him had appeared to be an asexual being and had never made any allusion to such a forbidden topic throughout the treatment, was now in the throes of an hysterical childbirth . . . the logical termination of a phantom pregnancy that had been invisibly developing in response to Breuer's ministrations. Though profoundly shocked, he managed to calm her down by hypnotizing her, and then fled the house in a cold sweat. The next day he and his wife left for Venice to spend a second honeymoon, which resulted in the conception of a daughter.[5]

Se non è vero, è ben trovato. The point of the story was that Freud, nothing if not "Faustian," picked up the key and put it to use.

Breuer had been taken unawares when sexuality turned up in the clinical setting. Freud was determined that future therapists should be forewarned: they should be put on notice that their patients would fall in love with them. And it was not just a matter of some patients and some doctors; it happened in all cases irrespective of age. With regard to a "young girl and a youngish man," it was perfectly "understandable" that she "should fall in love with a man" with whom she could "be much alone and talk of intimate things" and who had "the advantage of having met her as a helpful superior." With regard to a "woman unhappy in her marriage," suddenly "seized with a serious passion for a doctor" (who was still unattached), "ready to seek divorce in order to be with him," or, if that was impossible, ready to "enter into a secret *liaison*," it would be more unusual, but such things did occur "even outside psycho-analysis." What, then, of cases where there were "positively grotesque incongruities," cases of elderly women falling in love with grey-bearded men, cases, in short, where in the world's judgment there was "nothing of any kind to entice"? Even "under the most unfavourable conditions," Freud insisted, "the affectionate attachment by the patient to the doctor" came "to light again and again."[6]

It happened irrespective of gender. With male patients "the same attachment to the doctor, the same overvaluation of his qualities, the same absorption in his interests, the same jealousy of everyone close to him in real life"—these sublimated forms of sexuality were amply apparent. "Straightforward sexual demands," Freud noted, might be rarer in men than in women; hostility, that is, sexuality with a negative sign, however, was more common.[7] It almost inevitably came to pass that one day the patient's "positive attitude towards the analyst" would change "over into the negative, hostile one."[8] Whether negative or positive, the patient's intense feelings threatened to render the analyst impotent.

That hostility should make the patient resistant to treatment was not surprising. That passionate affection should have a similar effect might be puzzling. When hostility gained the upper hand, the patient naturally forgot "the intentions with which he [had] started the treatment"; he disregarded "the logical arguments and conclusions which only a short time before had made a great impression on him";[9] therapeutic gains were "blown away like chaff before the wind."[10] In contrast, one might imagine that passion "would be favourable to . . .

analytic purposes."[11] Not so, said Freud. When passion held sway, the patient suddenly lost "all understanding of the treatment and all interest in it"; "her docility, her acceptance of . . . the analytic explanations, her remarkable comprehension and the high degree of intelligence" which she had earlier demonstrated were "swept away."[12] She became quite without insight and seemed to be swallowed up in a love that now grew exacting, calling for "affectionate and sensual satisfactions."[13]

What was to be done? The "well-educated layman," a figure whom Freud summoned up as interlocutor, might hope for a simple answer: the treatment must come to an end. The hostile patient would decamp; the passionate patient would be asked by the doctor himself to take her leave. No other course, such as marriage or an illicit love affair, was compatible with "conventional morality and professional standards."[14]

Freud had no intention of defying conventional morality and professional standards. The analyst, he emphasized, "must not derive any personal advantage" from a patient's falling in love.

> I do not mean to say that it is always easy for the doctor to keep within the limits prescribed by ethics. . . . Those who are youngish and not yet bound by strong ties may in particular find it a hard task. . . . Again, when a woman sues for love, to reject and refuse is a distressing part for a man to play; and, in spite of neurosis . . . there is an incomparable fascination in a woman of high principles who confesses her passion. It is not a patient's crudely sensual desires which constitute the temptation. . . . It is rather, perhaps, a woman's subtler and aim-inhibited wishes which bring with them the danger of making a man forget . . . his medical task for the sake of a fine experience.[15]

In 1883, writing to his fiancée about Breuer and Anna O., Freud had taken pains to reassure Martha that he would not be forgetful, that he would remain entirely hers—and that to suffer Frau Breuer's fate, one had to be the wife of Breuer.[16] He was not Breuer. He would neither succumb nor flee; he would stay on the sexually saturated battlefield which had become the locus of psychoanalysis.

·   ·   ·

At the end of 1892, that is, at the time Freud was at work with Elisabeth von R. and had come to expect scenes of emotional conflict to be associated with the onset of hysterical symptoms, Lucy R. visited him during his consulting hours. This new patient was a young Englishwoman employed as governess for the children of a factory director in Vienna. She could, Freud wrote, best be described as a "marginal" case of "pure hysteria," and an "unmistakable" instance not only of conflict, but of conflict derived from sexuality—"an unmistakable sexual aetiology." It was her nose that brought her to him: its interior "was completely analgesic and without reflexes"; and "the perception proper to it as a sense-organ was absent." At the same time she was almost continually pursued by a "subjective olfactory sensation"—the smell of burnt pudding.[17]

Freud started the treatment and started to hypnotize his patient, to no avail. As with Elisabeth, so now with Lucy, he discovered that his powers as hypnotist had "severe limits." Without hypnosis and the expansion of memory it produced, how would his patient gain access to the requisite scenes? He was encouraged by an experiment in which a hypnotist gave "a woman in a state of somnambulism a negative hallucination that he was no longer present and had then endeavoured to draw her attention to himself in a great variety of ways, including some of a decidedly aggressive kind." After she had been woken up and despite her denial that she knew what had gone on, he "insisted that she could remember everything and laid his hand on her forehead to help her to recall it. And lo and behold! she ended by describing" all that had occurred.[18] With this experiment in mind, Freud surmised that to abandon hypnosis, a step which had been thrust upon him, would not entail abandoning analysis.

"Concentration" combined with "pressure" took the place of hypnosis. Freud started once more, this time with the assumption that Lucy knew everything that "was of any pathogenic significance" and that his task was to oblige her to communicate what she knew. When she professed ignorance as to the origin of her hysterical symptom, he judged the failure to be one not of memory but of concentration. He told her to lie down, shut her eyes, and try again. Concentration in itself, however, might not be enough: recollecting might break off "after a few sentences."[19] Pressure had to be applied: Freud placed his hands on his patient's forehead or he took her head between them and enjoined her to think, assuring her that something would come into her head, something she should catch hold of because it would be precisely what they had been searching for.[20] In his role as hypnotist,

Freud's powers had proved intermittent. His new technique spared him embarrassment: his patient, not he, now had to perform.

Lucy began without further ado. She "lay quietly . . . with her eyes closed . . . her features somewhat rigid, and without moving hand or foot." In response to Freud's query about the occasion on which she first smelled the burnt pudding, she replied that she could see the scene as "large as life," just as she had "experienced it." The time: two months earlier, two days before her birthday; the place: the school-room; the dramatis personae: the two little girls who were her charges and herself. They were "playing at cooking" when a servant entered and handed her a letter with a Glasgow postmark, obviously from her mother. The children grabbed it from her, proclaiming that it must be for her birthday and that they would keep it for her until then.[21] In their excitement they forgot the pudding they had been cooking; it ended up burnt, and Lucy ended up pursued by its smell.

Lucy was equally forthcoming in answer to the questions Freud posed in order to discover what had been "agitating" in this scene. As it turned out, Lucy had been set on returning to her mother and leaving the children; it also turned out that her mother had not sent for her daughter nor expressed any need of her, whereas the children were affectionate and needed her very much. Lucy had promised their mother, a distant relation, "on her death-bed," that she would devote herself to them and that she "would take their mother's place." Why, then, Freud, asked, had she been planning to break this promise? Trouble below stairs was Lucy's reply: the housekeeper, the cook, and the French governess had intrigued against her, and she had not received the support from her employer that she had expected. And though she had given notice, she had been advised to "think the matter over for a couple of weeks."[22] Lucy had now placed the scene in context.

But why, Freud wondered, hadn't "these agitations and this conflict of affects . . . remained on the level of normal psychical life?" What was missing, he surmised on the basis of other cases such as those of Emmy and Elisabeth, was an idea which had to be defended against, an idea which was antithetic to or incompatible with "the dominant mass of ideas constituting the ego," and which had therefore been *"intentionally repressed from consciousness."* Putting together "her fondness for the children and her sensitiveness on the subject of the other members of the household," he could draw only one conclusion: Lucy was in love with her employer; she nourished hopes of actually becoming mother to the children; and she was afraid that the servants had some inkling of her feelings. Lucy confirmed the interpretation, prompting Freud to ask why she had not told him earlier:

"I didn't know—or rather I didn't want to know. I wanted to drive it out of my head and not think of it again; and I believe latterly I have succeeded." "Why was it that you were unwilling to admit this inclination? Were you ashamed of loving a man?"—"Oh no, I'm not unreasonably prudish."

In this instance what had rendered the idea incompatible was disparity in social station: Lucy was "only a poor girl," and her employer was "such a rich man of good family."[23]

The repression lifted. She described how her love had begun, how one day her employer, "whose behaviour towards her had always been reserved, began a discussion . . . on the lines along which children should be brought up. He unbent more and was more cordial than usual and told her how much he depended on her for looking after his orphaned children; and as he said this he looked at her meaningly." It had been an hour of "intimate exchange," and she had anticipated another, but in vain. "There was no prospect," she acknowledged to Freud, of her feelings for her employer "meeting with any return." After this intimate exchange with his patient Freud anticipated "a fundamental change in her condition"—also in vain. What happened instead was that the first subjective olfactory sensation gave way to a second: "the smell of burnt pudding . . . became less frequent and weaker" and finally disappeared; "a similar smell, resembling cigar-smoke," became noticeable. Lucy thought "it had been there earlier as well . . . but had, as it were, been covered by the smell of the pudding."[24] Freud, a notorious cigar-smoker, now set out to discover what this second subjective olfactory sensation was covering in its turn.

He applied pressure: with his hands on her forehead and with his verbal injunctions ringing in her ears, a scene gradually began to unfold before Lucy's closed eyes. The time: luncheon; the place: the dining room of the house in which she was employed; the dramatis personae: the children, their father and grandfather, the French governess, the housekeeper, and Lucy herself—after further effort another figure came into view, a guest, the elderly chief accountant. As they were getting up from the table and the children were saying good-bye, the accountant tried to kiss them. Lucy's employer flared up and shouted at him not to do so. Lucy felt a "stab" at her "heart," and a strong and enduring scent of cigar smoke (the gentlemen had been smoking) entered her nose.[25]

Here, then, Freud noted, "was a second and deeper-lying scene which, like the first, operated as a trauma and left a mnemic symbol behind"—it actually had occurred earlier. Yet he was not satisfied: he remained puzzled about why Lucy had experienced the scene as traumatic. After all, he commented to his patient, the director's reprimand had not been addressed to her. Perhaps, he suggested, it was her employer's violence that hurt Lucy; perhaps, he continued, she worried that if he could become so enraged about "such a small thing with an old friend and guest," what might he be like if she were his wife?[26] Lucy admitted that Freud was getting close: the stab she had felt had to do with the director's violence, but also with the children being kissed—something he had never liked.

Again Lucy submitted to Freud's pressure; again a scene emerged—the one which proved to be "the really operative trauma and which had given the scene with the chief accountant its traumatic effectiveness." The time: "a few months earlier still"; the place: the director's home; the dramatis personae: Lucy, the children, their father, and a lady. The lady kissed the children on the mouth and took her leave. The director's fury burst upon Lucy's head: "he held her responsible . . . she was guilty of a dereliction of duty . . . , if it ever happened again he would entrust his children's upbringing to other hands." This rebuke had been delivered just when Lucy was hoping for a further intimate exchange, and it had "crushed her hopes."[27]

Two days after narrating this scene Lucy returned for a final visit. Freud "examined her nose and found that its sensitivity to pain and reflex excitability had been almost completely restored. She was also able to distinguish between smells, though with uncertainty and only if they were strong." He inquired as well about a dramatic change of mood: her seemingly chronic low spirits and fatigue had dissipated, and a cheerful Lucy reported that she felt freed from a "great weight":

"And what do you think of your prospects in the house?"—"I am quite clear on the subject. I know I have none, and I shan't make myself unhappy over it." . . .—"And are you still in love with your employer?"— "Yes, I certainly am, but that makes no difference. . . . I can have thoughts and feelings to myself."[28]

Freud could not fail to recognize and appreciate this fundamental change in his patient's condition. What he did not recognize or appreciate was the sexual scene that had been enacted under his very nose. The time: the present; the place: his consulting room; the dramatis personae: Freud and Lucy.

.   .   .

Lucy's hysteria had been marginal. Dora's was *"petite."* It displayed merely "the commonest of all somatic and mental symptoms": her nervous cough and aphonia ranked as physical (dyspnoea and migraines had come and gone in her earlier medical history); "depression, hysterical unsociability, and a *tedium vitae*" figured as mental.[29] In both cases Freud detected an unmistakable sexual etiology, but it was equally clear that in the meantime "sexual etiology" had undergone a sea change. With Lucy—"an over-mature girl with a need to be loved, whose affections had been aroused through a misunderstanding"[30]— Freud had focused on psychical trauma and at the same time had expected something in the way of anxiety neurosis to turn up. (It had not.) With Dora he focused his attention on his patient's "infantile sexual activity." Anyone who knew "how to interpret the language of hysteria," he claimed, would in the course of a psychoanalysis discover that the neurosis itself derived from the patient's infantile sexuality, which had come to be repressed.[31]

How might that discovery be made? From Lucy to Dora, Freud wrote, psychoanalytic technique had been "completely revolutionized."[32] Here is a description of the new regime.

> Without exerting any . . . kind of influence, he [the analyst] invites them [the patients] to lie down in a comfortable attitude on a sofa, while he himself sits on a chair behind them outside their field of vision. He does not even ask them to close their eyes, and avoids touching them in any way, as well as any other procedure which might be reminiscent of hypnosis. The session thus proceeds like a conversation between two

people equally awake, but one of whom is spared every muscular exertion and every distracting sensory impression which might divert his attention from his own mental activity.[33]

It was no ordinary conversation. The patient was enjoined "to say everything that came into his head, even if it was *unpleasant* to him, or seemed *unimportant* or *irrelevant* or *senseless.*"[34] It was Frau Emmy von N. who had admonished Freud to allow the patient to take the lead. Early on she had rebuked him for asking her "where this or that came from" rather than letting her tell "what she had to say."[35] By the time Dora arrived in Freud's consulting room, Emmy's admonition was in the course of being transformed into the fundamental rule.

Between Lucy and Dora, Freud's notion of what to interpret was also in the course of being transformed. In 1892 his prime concern had been to fill in gaps: he had vigilantly pursued pathogenic memories, often first eliciting, by means of pressure on his patient's head, "an intermediate link" between the memory that served as the point of departure and the pathogenic quarry.[36] In 1900 he was still concerned with gaps; he still thought psychoanalysis might repair "damage to the patient's memory." But he now treated his patients' material with a suspicion he had not earlier displayed. Having recently completed *The Interpretation of Dreams* and being on the verge of drafting *The Psychopathology of Everyday Life,* he approached what Dora produced, be it a memory or "a sound and incontestable train of argument," as if it were the stuff that dreams were made of.[37]

As for dreams themselves, Freud eagerly seized the opportunity they offered to deploy his full complement of interpretive artillery. (Between Lucy and Dora, his patients, heeding his injunction to "communicate . . . every idea or thought that occurred to them in connection with some particular subject," had, among other things, told him their dreams.)[38] Recall Dora's first dream, the recurrent one. (Freud recorded its manifest content immediately after the session, and this text then anchored the "chain of interpretations and recollections" that followed.)[39] The associations Dora produced, coupled with Freud's interrogation, provided a wealth of material about her relationship with Herr K. and with her father, and about her childhood history of bedwettting. Thanks to Freud's continued interrogation, it also introduced Dora's mother, who had hitherto been relegated to the background, in part because the patient herself "looked down on her . . . and used to criticize her mercilessly, and . . . had withdrawn completely from her influence." Recall also the jewel-case that Dora's mother had wanted to save. Dora associated:

> "Mother is very fond of jewellery and had a lot given her by Father."
> "And you?"
> "I used to be fond of jewellery too, once; but I have not worn any since my illness.—Once, four years ago . . . , Father and Mother had a great dispute about a piece of jewellery. Mother wanted to be given a particular thing—pearl drops to wear in her ears. But Father does not like that kind of thing and he bought her a bracelet instead of the drops. She was furious, and told him that as he had spent so much money on a present she did not like he had better just give it to some one else."
> "I dare say you thought to yourself you would accept it with pleasure."
> "I don't know. [This, Freud footnoted, was "the regular formula with which she confessed to anything that had been repressed."][40] I don't in the least know how Mother comes into the dream. . . ."
> "You ask how she comes into the dream? She is, as you know, your former rival in your father's affections. In the incident of the bracelet, you would have been glad to accept what your mother had rejected. Now let us just put 'give' instead of 'accept' and 'withhold' instead of 'reject'. Then it means that you were ready to give your father what your mother withheld from him; and the thing in question was connected with jewellery."[41]

At this point Freud dropped Dora's mother. (The jewel-case served as the point of intersection of several associative chains, and he chose to pursue the link among jewelery, jewel-case, and Herr K. He claimed that Dora was afraid not only of Herr K., but of the temptation she felt "to yield to him." Dora demurred.)[42]

Freud was obliged to pick up where he had left off. The dream itself deserved to rank as an event; it had sequelae in waking life that demanded interpretation. For several days after work on it, Dora "identified herself with her mother by means of slight symptoms and peculiarities of manner, which gave her an opportunity for some really remarkable achievements in the direction of intolerable behaviour." She then told how her mother had suffered from abdominal pains and from a vaginal discharge ("a catarrh") and how in Dora's view—and Freud thought "she was probably right"—her mother's illness "was due to her father, who had . . . handed on his venereal disease. . . ." (The father apparently had had gonorrhea as well as syphilis. About the latter, Dora was well informed.) The "persistence" with which Dora identified with her mother, coupled with this information, led Freud "to ask her whether she too was suffering from a venereal disease"; she admitted to being "afflicted with a catarrh (leucorrhoea)" whose onset "she could not remember."[43]

> She had learnt to call her affection a "catarrh" at the time when her mother had had . . . a similar complaint, and the word "catarrh" acted . . . as a "switch-word," and enabled the whole set of thoughts upon her father's responsibility for her illness to manifest themselves in the symptom of the cough . . . , which no doubt originated . . . from a slight actual catarrh. . . . It proclaimed aloud, as it were, something of which she may have been still unconscious: "I am my father's daughter. . . . He has made me ill, just as he has made Mother ill. It is from him that I have got my evil passions, which are punished by illness."[44]

At this point Freud dropped Dora's father. (He fastened on the disease instead. Leukorrhea as well as bedwetting, he thought, pointed to masturbation—he later changed his mind about leukorrhea. Dora's "premature sexual enjoyment and its consequences," he argued, addressing his readers, not his patient, had led to a repudiation of sexuality, to her falling "ill of a neurosis," and to her inability "to yield to her love" for Herr K.)[45]

Once again Freud was obliged to pick up where he had left off, thanks to a second dream, which Dora reported a few weeks after the first. Here is the dream:

> *"I was walking about in a town which I did not know. . . . Then I came into a house where I lived, went to my room, and found a letter from mother lying there. She wrote saying that as I had left home without my parents' knowledge she had not wished to write to me to say that Father was ill. "Now he is dead, and if you like you can come." I then went to the station [Bahnhof] and asked about a hundred times: "Where is the station?" I always got the answer: "Five minutes." I then saw a thick wood before me which I went into, and there I asked a man whom I met. He said to me: "Two and a half hours more." He offered to accompany me. But I refused and went alone. I saw the station in front of me and could not reach it. I had the usual feeling of anxiety that one has in dreams when one cannot*

120

move forward. Then I was at home. . . . The maidservant opened the door to me and replied that Mother and the others were already at the cemetery [Friedhof].[46]

In interpreting this dream Freud was obliged to notice Dora's hostility to her father. After all, its subject was his death. The words *"she asked quite a hundred times"* led Dora to voice concern about her father's health: she recalled having been asked by him, the evening before the dream, for some brandy to help him sleep; she in turn had asked her mother, she exclaimed impatiently, *"a hundred times"* for the key to the sideboard. And the words *"contents of the letter"* led Freud to associate to a suicide note Dora had written, which, he had surmised, had aimed at frightening her father (and which in fact had prompted him to bring her for treatment). The manifest content itself suggested that "she had left home and gone among strangers, and her father's heart had broken with grief and with longing for her"—a fantasy which Freud interpreted as one of revenge. Having noted "Dora's *craving for revenge,*" he let the matter drop.[47]

Instead, Freud concentrated on what had puzzled him (and what by this time had also come to puzzle Dora) about the famous scene by the lake. Dora recognized the phrase in the letter "if you like," to which she appended a question mark, "as a quotation out of the letter from Frau K." inviting her for the fateful visit. Once again Freud asked her to describe the scene. To escape Herr K., after slapping him, Dora had first thought of walking round the lake, and *"she had asked a man whom she met how far it was."* He had replied: *"Two and a half hours,"* and so she had taken the boat. The *"wood"* in the dream was like the wood by the shore of the lake and like the wood where Herr K. had propositioned her. And Dora had seen the same thick wood the day before in a picture at an exhibition, a picture that included nymphs as well as woods. At this point a "suspicion" of Freud's turned into a "certainty"—and he informed his patient of that certainty:

The use of *Bahnhof* [station; literally, railway-court] and *Friedhof* [cemetery; literally, peace-court] to represent the female genitals was striking enough in itself. . . . But now, with the addition of "nymphs" visible in the background of a "thick wood," no further doubts could be entertained. Here was a symbolic geography of sex! "Nymphae," as is known to physicians . . . is the name given to the labia minora, which lie in the background of the "thick wood" of the pubic hair. . . . There lay concealed behind the . . . situation in the dream a phantasy of defloration, the phantasy of a man seeking to force entrance into the female genitals.[48]

The interpretation, Freud surmised, must have made a "forcible . . . impression." Dora now recalled an attack of appendicitis, more precisely an attack occurring nine months after Herr K.'s proposition. Here, Freud told his patient, was a fantasy of childbirth.

> "If it is true that you were delivered of a child nine months after the scene by the lake, . . . then it follows that in your unconscious you must have regretted the upshot of the scene. . . . So you see that your love for Herr K. did not come to an end with the scene, but that (as I maintained) it has persisted down to the present day—though it is true you are unconscious of it."

Freud was satisfied, if not triumphant, not least of all because "Dora disputed the fact no longer."[49]

His satisfaction proved short-lived. Dora began the next session—December 31, 1900—with the following words:

> "Do you know that I am here for the last time to-day?"—"How can I know, as you have said nothing to me about it?"—"Yes. I made up my mind to put up with it till the New Year. But I shall wait no longer than that to be cured."—"You know that you are free to stop the treatment at any time. But for to-day we will go on with our work."

That work proceeded with Freud asking Dora when she had reached her decision. Her reply—a fortnight ago—brought to his mind the image of a maidservant or governess giving notice. And "governess" prompted Dora to give at last a full account of what had occurred during her visit to the Ks. Her hosts had had a governess in their employ. Herr K., so the young woman had confided to Dora, had seduced her, and when it became clear that he was also going to abandon her, she had given notice. Herr K., so Dora confided to Freud in turn, had used to her the very phrases that he had earlier addressed to the governess. Freud interpreted:

> "'Does he dare,' you said to yourself, 'to treat me like a governess, like a servant?' Wounded pride added to jealousy, and to the conscious motives of common sense—it was too much. . . . You told your parents

what happened—a fact which we have hitherto been unable to account for. . . ."

"It must have been a bitter piece of disillusionment for you when the effect of your charge against Herr K. was not that he renewed his proposals but that he replied instead with denials. . . . You will agree that nothing makes you so angry as having it thought that you merely fancied the scene by the lake. I know now—and this is what you do not want to be reminded of—that you *did* fancy that Herr K.'s proposals were serious, and that he would not leave off until you had married him."

Dora listened "without any of her usual contradictions. She seemed moved; she said good-bye . . . very warmly, with the heartiest wishes for the New Year, and—came no more."[50]

Her announcement that she was breaking off treatment struck Freud as a nasty surprise; it struck him just when his "hopes of a successful termination . . . were at their highest." He consoled himself with the reflection that any one who conjured up "the most evil of those half-tamed demons that inhabit the human breast" and sought "to wrestle with them" should be prepared for reverses.[51] After all, as early as *Studies on Hysteria* he had recognized that he—and his then much-prized pressure technique—risked defeat if those half-tamed demons, that is, "distressing ideas" arising "from the content of the analysis," were "transferred on to the figure of the physician." He had given an example:

> In one of my patients the origin of a particular hysterical symptom lay in a wish, which she had had many years earlier and had at once relegated to the unconscious, that the man she was talking to at the time might boldly take the initiative and give her a kiss. On one occasion, at the end of a session, a similar wish came up in her about me. She was horrified at it, spent a sleepless night, and at the next session, though she did not refuse to be treated, was quite useless for work. After I had discovered the obstacle and removed it, the work proceeded further.[52]

In the postscript to Dora's case, in an effort to account for its abrupt termination, Freud spelled out at greater length what he meant by transferences.

> What are transferences? They are new editions or facsimiles of the impulses and phantasies which are aroused and made conscious during the progress of the analysis; but they have this peculiarity, which is charac-

teristic for their species, that they replace some earlier person by the person of the physician. To put it another way: a whole series of psychological experiences are revived, not as belonging to the past, but as applying to the person of the physician at the present moment. Some of these transferences have a content which differs from that of their model in no respect whatever except for the substitution. These then—to keep to the same metaphor—are merely new impressions or reprints. Others are more ingeniously contructed; their content has been subjected to a moderating influence . . . and they may even become conscious, by cleverly taking advantage of some real peculiarity in the physician's person or circumstances and attaching themselves to that. These, then, will no longer be new impressions, but revised editions.[53]

Of whom was Freud a new or a revised edition? Dora had offered him a clue in the form of a forgotten memory appended to the first dream. After waking from the most recent occurrence of this recurrent dream, she reported, she "had smelt smoke," and "she thought, too, that she clearly remembered having noticed the smell of smoke on the . . . occasions" she had dreamt the dream before fleeing the Alpine lake with her father. Smoke obviously referred to the dream's manifest content—a house was on fire; it also referred to Herr K. and her father, both of whom, she reported, were "passionate smokers"; it less obviously referred to Dora's analyst:

The addendum . . . could scarcely mean anything else than the longing for a kiss, which, with a smoker, would necessarily smell of smoke. But a kiss had passed between Herr K. and Dora some two years further back, and it would certainly have been repeated more than once if she had given way to him. . . . Taking into consideration, finally, the indications which seemed to point to there having been a transference on to me— since I am a smoker too—I came to the conclusion that the idea had probably occurred to her one day during a session that she would like to have a kiss from me.[54]

Freud did not communicate his interpretation to Dora. (He thought that there was no pressing need. He thought of transferences as something that blocked access to memories, and at this point in the treatment "the material for the analysis had not yet run dry.")[55] In retrospect he realized what he should have done then:

When the first dream came, in which she gave herself the warning that she had better leave my treatment just as she had formerly left Herr K.'s house, I ought to have listened to the warning myself. "Now," I ought to have said to her, "it is from Herr K. that you have made a transference on to me. Have you noticed anything that leads you to suspect me of evil intentions similar . . . to Herr K.'s? Or have you been struck by anything about me or got to know anything about me which has caught your fancy, as happened previously with Herr K.?" Her attention would then have been turned to some detail . . . behind which there lay concealed something analogous but immeasurably more important concerning Herr K.

And so, Freud was confident, he would have succeeded "in mastering the transference in good time."[56]

.   .   .

"An unknown quantity" in him, Freud argued, "had reminded Dora of Herr K."[57] Only of Herr K.?[58] At the beginning of the treatment Dora consciously and constantly compared Freud with her father. In presenting her history, Freud emphasized his patient's longstanding, tender paternal attachment. In recapitulating his interpretation of her first dream, he insisted that Dora was summoning up "her infantile affection for her father . . . in order to protect herself against . . . love" for Herr K. In interpreting her second dream, he noted Dora's hostility to her father, but did not pursue it. (Nor did he consider that it might also have been longstanding.) In retrospect Freud reviewed that second dream, picking out particular elements which taken together led to a summary statement of Dora's latent dream thoughts: "Men are all so detestable that I would rather not marry. This is my revenge." Without mentioning her father, without hinting at a possible transference from him, Freud concluded that during treatment the physician had become the target of Dora's "cruel impulses and revengeful motives." And he wondered, "how could the patient take a more effective revenge than by demonstrating on her own person" his "helplessness and incapacity," that is, by not getting well?[59]

In 1920 Freud published a paper entitled "The Psychogenesis of a Case of Homosexuality in a Woman" that can be read as an addendum to the one on Dora. (Recall his cursory reference to Dora's love for Frau K. In a footnote to the postscript he reproached himself for his failure "to discover in time and to inform the patient that her homosexual [gynaecophilic] love for Frau K. was the strongest unconscious current in her mental life.")[60] As with Dora, so too with an unnamed "beautiful and clever girl of eighteen," it was a father who brought his daughter for treatment. The father was outraged by the "devoted adoration with which she pursued" a woman ten years her senior, who was known to be having "intimate relations" with a married woman, while at the same time carrying on "promiscuous affairs with a number of men." This "one interest had swallowed up all others in the girl's mind." She neglected her education and "thought nothing of social functions or girlish pleasures." Freud appreciated, as he had not when Dora had been brought to him, that it was "not a matter of indifference" whether someone came to analysis of her own accord or because she was taken to it—whether it was she or her relatives who wanted her to change. He also appreciated that "to convert a fully developed homosexual into a heterosexual" did not "offer much more prospect of success than the reverse, except that for good practical reasons the latter" was "never attempted." Still he "was prepared to study the girl carefully for a few weeks or months, so as then to be able to pronounce how far a continuation of the analysis would be likely to influence her."[61]

That careful study or preliminary phase—a number of analyses, Freud noted, fell into "two clearly distinguishable phases"—allowed him to "obtain an adequate insight . . . into the way in which her inversion had developed." About her childhood, he unearthed nothing pertinent: "she could not remember any sexual traumas in early life, nor were any discovered by analysis"; she did not show any signs of having engaged in "infantile masturbation," nor did the analysis "throw any light on this point"; she did pass through the "normal attitude" of being strongly attached to her father. "During the prepubertal years at school she gradually became acquainted with the facts of sex, and she received this knowledge with mixed feelings of lasciviousness and frightened aversion"—again a thoroughly normal response. Shortly after puberty, at the age of thirteen or fourteen, she had shown marked affection for a small boy, and Freud inferred that she was then "possessed of a strong desire to be a mother herself and to have a child." At about sixteen a small boy actually entered her own family—a baby brother. Thereupon "she became a homosexual attracted to mature women, and remained so every since."[62] ("Her genital chastity," however, Freud was happy to learn, was "intact.")[63]

Thanks to "a series of dreams, interrelated and easy to interpret," he felt confident that his account of his patient's sexual reorientation was not a product of his "inventive powers."

> It was just when the girl was experiencing the revival of her infantile Oedipus complex at puberty that she suffered her great disappointment. She became keenly conscious of the wish to have a child, and a male one; that what she desired was her *father's* child and an image of *him*, her consciousness was not allowed to know. And what happened next? It was not *she* who bore the child, but her unconsciously hated rival, her mother. Furiously resentful and embittered, she turned away from her father and from men altogether. After this first great reverse she foreswore her womanhood and sought another goal for her libido.[64]

The girl's relation to her father, then, had been of decisive importance in her sexual history; it "had the same decisive importance for the course and outcome of the analytic treatment, or rather, analytic exploration." The girl transferred on to Freud "the same sweeping repudiation of men which had dominated her ever since the disappointment she had suffered from her father." "As soon . . . as I recognized the girl's attitude to her father, I broke off the treatment and advised her parents that if they set store by the therapeutic procedure it should be continued by a woman doctor." This time Freud was less confident that he could succeed "in mastering the transference in good time." "Bitterness against men is as a rule easy to gratify upon the physician; it need not evoke any violent emotional manifestations, it simply expresses itself by rendering futile all his endeavours and by clinging to the illness."[65]

"The Chief Patient"

"The chief patient I am preoccupied with is myself. . . . The analysis is more difficult than any other. . . . Still, I believe it must be done and is a necessary intermediate stage in my work."[66] So Freud wrote Fliess on August 14, 1897. When had he become his own chief patient? When did he relinquish that role? How did he conduct the treatment? The answer to the first question is clear: summer 1897. The answer to the second has eluded scholars, though no one has suggested a terminal date prior to 1900; so too has an answer to a related query of whether the self-analysis was intermittent or continuous, though intermittent is more plausible. As for its mode of conduct, all are agreed that dream interpretation ranked as the principal means and that "traces of the experience" found their way into Freud's dream book.[67]

Here is the first dream he "submitted to a detailed interpretation":

> *A large hall—numerous guests, whom we were receiving.—Among them was Irma. I at once took her on one side, as though to answer her letter and to reproach her for not having accepted my "solution" yet. I said to her: "If you still get pains, it's really only your fault." She replied: "If you only knew what pains I've got now in my throat and stomach and abdomen—it's choking me"—I was alarmed and looked at her. She looked pale and puffy. I thought to myself that after all I must be missing some organic trouble. I took her to the window and looked down her throat, and she showed signs of recalcitrance, like women with artificial dentures. I thought to myself that there was really no need for her to do that.—She then opened her mouth properly and on the right I found a big white patch; at another place I saw extensive whitish grey scabs upon some remarkable curly structures which were evidently modelled on the turbinal bones of the nose.—I at once called in Dr. M., and he repeated the examination and confirmed it. . . . Dr. M. looked quite different from usual; he was very pale, he walked with a limp and his chin was clean-shaven. . . . My friend Otto was now standing beside her as well, and my friend Leopold was percussing her through her bodice and saying: "She has a dull area on the left." He also indicated that a portion of the skin on the left shoulder was infiltrated. (I noticed this, just as he did, in spite of her dress.) . . . M. said: "There's no doubt it's an infection, but no matter; dysentery will supervene and the toxin will be eliminated." . . . We were directly aware, too, of the origin of the infection. Not long before, when she was feeling unwell, my friend Otto had given her an injection of a preparation of propyl, propyls . . . propionic acid . . . trimethylamin (and I saw before me the formula for this printed in heavy type). . . . Injections of that sort ought not to be made so thoughtlessly. . . . And probably the syringe had not been clean.[68]*

The evening before the dream, Freud's friend Otto, also a physician, had brought him news of Irma, a former patient, whose psychoanalytic treatment had ended with only a qualified success: she had been relieved of her "hysterical anxiety" but not of "all her somatic symptoms." In Otto's report—"she's better, but not quite well"—Freud discerned a reproach: he had promised too much and delivered too little. To justify himself, he sat down that same evening "to write out Irma's case history," with the idea of sending it to Dr. M., the leading figure in his and Otto's medical circle. Given this background information alone, Freud argued, one would not "have the slightest notion of what the dream meant."[69] Given the dream's manifest content, however, it was obvious that the case history had continued to trouble him in his sleep.

He took as his point of departure his initial diagnosis of hysteria. If Irma's pains were hysterical, he mused, was it not his responsibility to relieve them? Yes and no. In his view, at the time he dreamt the dream, that responsibility extended only to the point of informing his patient of the hidden meaning of her symptom, that is, of solving the symptom's riddle. It did not extend to inducing the patient to accept the proffered solution—despite the fact that he considered recovery dependent upon such an acceptance. Hence if Irma's pains were hysterical, and if he had accurately divined their meaning and conveyed that meaning to her, she, not he, must bear the responsibility: *"If you still get pains, it's really only your fault."* Was blaming Irma the only way to avoid blaming himself?

He started over again. Pains in her *"throat and stomach and abdomen"*—these were not pains Irma had complained of; and *"pale and puffy"* did not describe her looks. Perhaps he had missed *"some organic trouble."* If that were so, Irma ought not to be rebuked. Should he? Initially he was prepared to answer in the negative; after all, his "treatment only set out to get rid of *hysterical* pains."

> *I took her to the window and looked down her throat, and she showed signs of recalcitrance, like women with artificial dentures.*

And when he examined the throat, what he saw—*"extensive whitish grey scabs upon some remarkable curly structures which were evidently modelled on the turbinal bones of the nose"*—reminded him of other figures and other scenes. He associated to his use of cocaine "to reduce some troublesome nasal swellings"; he recalled the fatal consequences of his recommending the drug to a friend; he recalled the fatal consequences of his "repeatedly prescribing" to a patient "what was at that time regarded as a harmless remedy (sulphonal)."[70] Freud was on the verge of incriminating himself.

He continued in pursuit of both the organic complaint and the responsible party. Irma faded out, leaving her body behind; medical colleagues appeared upon the scene, Dr. M. and Otto among them.

After examining the patient, Dr. M. remarked: *"There's no doubt it's an infection, but no matter; dysentery will supervene and the toxin will be eliminated."*

Dysentery struck Freud as a bizarre prognosis. Could it be, he wondered, that he "was trying to make fun of Dr. M.'s fertility in producing far-fetched explanations and making unexpected pathological connections?" He recalled an amusing story Dr. M. had once told of a consultation about a seriously ill patient: "He had felt obliged to point out, in view of the very optimistic view taken by his colleague, that he had found albumen in the patient's urine. The other [doctor], however, was not in the least put out: *'No matter,'* he had said, 'the albumen will soon be eliminated!'" Freud wondered no longer: he was taking revenge on Dr. M.—who had not agreed with the "solution" Freud had offered Irma—by showing that his senior colleague was "an ignoramus." Dysentery also reminded Freud of a young male patient who had had "remarkable difficulties associated with defaecating."

> I had recognized it as a hysteria, but had been unwilling to try him with my psychotherapeutic treatment and had sent him on a sea voyage. Some days before, I had had a despairing letter from him from Egypt, saying that he had had a fresh attack there which a doctor had declared was dysentery. I suspected that the diagnosis was an error on the part of an ignorant practitioner who had allowed himself to be taken in by the hysteria. But I could not help reproaching myself for having put my patient in a situation in which he might have contracted some organic trouble on top of his hysterical intestinal disorder.[71]

Once again Freud was on the verge of incriminating himself.

The source of Irma's pains—an infection—had been agreed upon along the way, and finally the culprit was identified:

> *We were directly aware, too, of the origin of the infection. Not long before, when she was feeling unwell, my friend Otto had given her an injection of a preparation of propyl. . . . Injections of that sort ought not to be made so thoughtlessly. . . . And probably the syringe had not been clean.*

Here Freud never doubted what he was trying to do: he was directly accusing Otto of thoughtlessness—and his associations continued in that vein. Further associations led him back to his dead friend and his dead patient; indirectly, then, he was accusing himself as well. He might list instances of his conscientiousness—he took great pains, he noted, to use clean syringes—but instances of the reverse outnumbered them. If the wish that had motivated the dream was exoneration, its fulfillment was far from complete.

One element in the manifest content, trimethylamin, stood out in heavy type—a sign that it possessed "a high degree of psychical significance."[72] Trimethylamin, Freud had been led to believe, was a product of sexual metabolism, and from there he associated to "the chemistry of the sexual processes." And so he arrived at his postulate of a sexual etiology for anxiety neurosis. (His "Reply to Criticisms of My Paper on Anxiety Neurosis" was published the same month he dreamt of Irma.) Like Emmy von N., Irma might well have fitted into the category of "intentionally abstinent people"; she was a young widow, and if Freud "wanted to find an excuse" for his treatment's failure, "the fact of her widowhood" best met the requirement.[73] Here was a diagnosis that fulfilled his wish to be exonerated. Trimethylamin also represented, as Freud admitted in 1908, his "sexual megalomania": "the one therapy for widowhood," for Irma and two other young widows—and he had "them all!"[74]

Trimethylamin alluded "to the immensely powerful factor of sexuality"; it also alluded to the friend with whom Freud had discussed sexual chemistry, a friend "whose agreement" Freud "recalled with satisfaction" whenever he "felt isolated."[75] And he had felt isolated and reproached—by Dr. M. as well as by Otto. Take Dr. M., that is, Breuer, away, so Freud's wish ran; give him instead his friend, that is, Fliess.

Freud reviewed the dream. He returned to the curly structures in Irma's throat that were modeled on the turbinal bones of the nose. Here he found another allusion to Fliess, an otolaryngologist who had drawn "scientific attention to . . . connections between the turbinal bones" and the female sex organs.[76] On Freud's urging Fliess had examined Irma to see whether, in her case, there was a link between her nose and her somatic symptoms. On Freud's urging his friend had also examined and then proceeded to operate on Emma Eckstein's nose—with nearly fatal consequences.[77] Given the dream's manifest content, it was obvious that Emma's case as well as Irma's continued to trouble Freud in his sleep.

Like Elisabeth von R., Emma suffered from "weakness in walking."[78] Beyond that the exact nature of her complaints is difficult to determine: severe menstrual bleeding and headaches, possibly migraines, crop up in Freud's correspondence with Fliess.[79] The weakness in walking Freud would have regarded as within his bailiwick; the severe bleeding would have prompted him to call in Fliess. In late January 1895 he wrote his friend:

> Now only one more week separates us from the operation, or at least from the preparations for it. . . . My lack of medical knowledge . . . weighs heavily on me. But I keep repeating to myself: so far as I have some insight into the matter, the cure must be achievable by this route. I would not have dared to invent this plan of treatment on my own, but I confidently join you in it.[80]

Fliess came to Vienna sometime during the first half of February, performed the operation, and left almost immediately. Freud's confidence turned out to have been misplaced.

Emma's condition, like Irma's, was "still unsatisfactory . . ." In early March Freud sent Fliess the following bulletin:

> The purulent secretion has been decreasing since yesterday; the day before yesterday . . . she had a massive hemorrhage, probably as a result of expelling a bone chip . . . there were two bowls full of pus. Today we encountered resistance on irrigation; and since the pain and visible edema had increased, I let myself be persuaded to call in Gersuny.

Like Dr. M. in the dream, the well-known plastic surgeon Robert Gersuny *"repeated the examination"*: "He explained that the access was considerably narrowed and insufficient for drainage, inserted a drainage tube, and threatened to break it [the bone?] open if that did not stay in. To judge by the smell, all this is most likely correct."[81] Gersuny had found something resembling an *"infection"* and certainly hoped that the *"toxin"* would be eliminated. In this instance *"dysentery"* would have come as a relief to one and all.

Instead, Emma had an even more massive hemorrhage. Here is Freud's report:

> Two days later I was awakened in the morning—profuse bleeding had started again, pain, and so on. Gersuny replied on the phone that he was unavailable till evening; so I asked [Ignaz] Rosanes to meet me. He did so at noon. There still was moderate bleeding from the nose and mouth; the fetid odor was very bad. Rosanes cleaned the area surrounding the opening, removed some sticky blood clots, and suddenly pulled at something like a thread, kept on pulling. Before either of us had time to think,

at least half a meter of gauze had been removed from the cavity. The next moment came a flood of blood. The patient turned white, her eyes bulged, and she had no pulse. Immediately thereafter, however, he again packed the cavity with fresh iodoform gauze and the hemorrhage stopped. . . . At the moment the foreign body came out and everything became clear to me—and I immediately afterward was confronted by the sight of the patient—I felt sick. After she had been packed, I fled to the next room, drank a bottle of water, and felt miserable.[82]

The source of Emma's "pains" had been tracked down; the pursuit of the responsible party began.

Was Fliess without blemish? He had accidentally left half a meter of iodoform gauze in the cavity created by the removal of the turbinal bone and the opening of a sinus, and he himself feared censure. For his "rehabilitation" he deemed "it necessary to have a testimonial certificate from Gersuny"; it was not forthcoming. (Recall how in his dream Freud portrayed Dr. M. as an "ignoramus.") For his part, Freud was ready to bear witness:

I have worked it through by now. I was not sufficiently clear at that time to think of immediately reproaching Rosanes. It only occurred to me . . . later that he should immediately have thought, There is something inside; I shall not pull it out lest there be a hemorrhage; rather, I'll stuff it [the cavity] some more, take her to [Sanatorium] Loew, and there clean and widen it at the same time.[83]

(Recall how in his dream Freud condemned Otto for proceeding "thoughtlessly.") The trimethylamin completed the rehabilitation of Fliess: it represented Freud's own work on the sexual etiology of anxiety neurosis as well as his friend's research on sex and the nose, a project Freud was certain would demonstrate Fliess's hold on "a beautiful piece of objective truth."[84]

Freud dreamt his dream of Irma on July 23–24, 1895, and interpreted it the following day.[85] But he did not communicate the dream and its interpretation to his friend immediately. In all likelihood he did not tell him of it until late autumn of 1897, that is, until he had had a few months experience as his own "chief patient."[86] He did not communicate it until he was beginning to suspect that "true self-analysis" was "impossible."[87] Was he enlisting for his analytic venture the physician he had described as "the type of man into whose hands one confidently puts one's life"? Was he enlisting the physician to whom he had written longingly the morning after the Irma dream?

> Daimonie [Demon], why don't you write? How are you? Don't you care at all any more about what I am doing? What is happening to the nose, menstruation, labor pain, neuroses . . . ? True, this year I am ill [Freud was suffering from cardiac symptoms] and must come to you; what will happen if by chance both of us remain healthy for a whole year? Are we friends only in misfortune? Or do we also want to share the experiences of calm times with each other?[88]

Was Freud's crypto-therapist also an object of his "sexual megalomania"?[89]

.   .   .

At Christmas time 1897 Freud and Fliess held a "congress" in Breslau. That same year Fliess's work, anticipated in the Irma dream, *Die Beziehungen zwischen Nase und weiblichen Geschlechtsorganen* (The Relations between the Nose and the Female Sexual Organs), had appeared in print. In the early 1890s Fliess had been preoccupied with, and had published on, pathological conditions of the nose. To such conditions he had attributed a myriad of symptoms including "disturbances in the general functioning of the cardiac, respiratory, gastric, and reproductive systems." By 1897 the link between the nose and the female menstrual cycle had led him to "vital periodicities manifested by all physiological processes," that is, to 28- and 23-day cycles.[90] By the time he met Freud in Breslau, periodicity theory in its turn had led him to the essential bisexuality of human beings.[91]

For his part, a few months before he met his friend in Breslau, Freud had discarded the seduction hypothesis and was confronted with the problem of establishing a new etiology for the defense neuroses. His famous letter confessing his loss of confidence in his *"neurotica"* was soon followed by another in which he mentioned his discovery of a "universal event in early childhood": "being in love" with mother and "jealous" of father. And just days before setting out he imparted his latest insight: "Masturbation is the one major habit, the 'primary addiction,' and it is only as a substitute and replacement for it that the other addictions—to alcohol, morphine, tobacco, and the like—come into existence. The role played by this addiction in hysteria is enormous."[92] Freud was taking the first steps toward his etiological goal.

He was also taking the first steps toward the dream book. In the same letter to Fliess admitting his doubts about seduction, he had consoled himself with the following reflection: "In this collapse of everything valuable, the psychological alone has remained untouched. The dream [book] stands entirely secure. . . . It is a pity one cannot make a living . . . on dream interpretation!" Within weeks of the Breslau meeting, Freud told his friend that he was "deep in the dream book, . . . writing it fluently," and enjoying "the thought of all the 'head-shaking'" over its "indiscretions and audacities." He also announced his intention of first exhibiting those indiscretions and audacities to Fliess: he proposed to send him the manuscript, in fragments, before he sent it to his publisher and begged him to perform "the duties of . . . supreme judge."[93]

On March 8 or 9, 1898, Freud received a letter from his friend: "I am very much occupied with your dream book. *I see it lying finished before me and I see myself turning over the pages.*"[94] On March 10 Freud replied:

> It was no small feat on your part to see the dream book lying before you. It has come to a halt again, and meanwhile the problem has deepened and widened. . . . Dream life seems to me to derive entirely from the residues of the prehistoric period of life (between the ages of one and three)—the same period which is the source of the unconscious and alone contains the etiology of all the psychoneuroses, the period normally characterized by an amnesia analogous to hysterical amnesia. . . . The repetition of what was experienced in that period is in itself the fulfillment of a wish; a recent wish only leads to a dream if it can put itself in connection with material from this prehistoric period, if the recent wish is a derivative of a prehistoric one or can get itself adopted by one.[95]

The dream that best fitted Freud's theorizing had been dreamt on an intervening night: it was the dream of the botanical monograph.[96]

In the course of the day following the dream Freud found no time to interpret it; he found time, however, to indulge in a daydream:

> If ever I got glaucoma, I had thought, I should travel to Berlin and get myself operated on, incognito, in my friend's [Fliess's] house, by a surgeon recommended by him. The operating surgeon, who would have

no idea of my identity, would boast once again of how easily such operations could be performed since the introduction of cocaine; and I should not give the slightest hint that I myself had had a share in the discovery.

Fliess alone would recognize the patient. (In 1884 Freud had published a "monograph" on the coca plant which had drawn Dr. Karl Koller's attention to the anesthetic properties of cocaine, and for exploiting that suggestion Koller had earned considerable renown—much to Freud's chagrin.) A recollection followed:

> Shortly after Koller's discovery, my father had in fact been attacked by glaucoma; my friend Dr. Königstein, the ophthalmic surgeon, had operated on him; while Dr. Koller had been in charge of the cocaine anaesthesia and had commented on the fact that this case had brought together all of the three men who had had a share in the introduction of cocaine.[97]

With the daydream and memory in mind he proceeded to interpret his dream.

Subsequently, he gave three versions of it:

> 1) *I had written a* MONOGRAPH *on a certain* (indistinct) *species of plant.*
> 2) *I had written a monograph on a certain plant. The book lay before me and I was at the moment turning over a folded coloured plate. Bound up in each copy was a dried specimen of the plant, as though it had been taken from a herbarium.*
> 3) *I had written a monograph on an (unspecified) genus of plants. The book lay before me and I was at the moment turning over a folded coloured plate. Bound up in the copy was a dried specimen of the plant.*[98]

He began his analysis by recalling an event of the preceding day which had turned up in the dream: the previous morning he had seen a new work "in the window of a book-shop, bearing the title *The Genus Cyclamen*—evidently a *monograph* on that plant."[99] The event itself was both recent and indifferent, yet it linked up with a far from indifferent conversation Freud had had the previous evening with Dr. Leopold Königstein. It also linked up with a series of memories. Botanical references forged the links. If such references had been absent from the stirring conversation or the series of memories, Freud argued, the dream would simply not have been the same: another indifferent impression would have served to represent them in the manifest content.

Freud arrived at the series of memories by way of associations to the *"folded coloured plate."* Initially he recalled how as a medical student, despite his limited means, he had managed to get hold of medical societies' proceedings and had been "enthralled by their coloured plates." A recollection from childhood followed:

> It had once amused my father to hand over a book with *coloured plates* (an account of a journey through Persia) for me and my eldest sister to destroy. Not easy to justify from the educational point of view! I had been five years old at the time and my sister not yet three; and the picture of the two of us blissfully pulling the book to pieces (leaf by leaf, like an *artichoke,* I found myself saying) was almost the only plastic memory that I retained from that period of my life.[100]

Freud did not interpret this scene as pointing to childhood sexual activities, any more than he did the screen memory of the green meadow and yellow flowers to which he referred when he was finishing *The Interpretation of Dreams* in 1899. Nor did he question the accuracy of the memory: that Jacob Freud, a self-taught man with a great respect for learning, would have allowed his children to tear up an illustrated book is hard to believe. The unlikelihood of this event, however, expressed in "plastic" form Freud's wish for an indulgent father.

The image faded. The father had not been amused when at the age of seventeen his son had run up "a largish account at the bookseller's" and had had "nothing to meet it with"; the father had not been amused by the son's defense that "his inclinations might have chosen a worse outlet." Further associations to roughly the same age followed. Freud recalled being asked by his headmaster, who displayed little confidence in his helpfulness, to clean the school's *"herbarium"*: "some small *worms*—book-worms—had found their way into it." Once again, Freud, a bookworm, was brought back to the bibliophile outlet his inclinations had chosen. He also recalled how on a preliminary botany examination he had failed to identify a "crucifer." From the Cruciferae he went on to the Compositae, and it occurred to him that artichokes—his favorite flowers—belonged to that genus. "Favorite" led him once more to his "bibliophile propensities": as a student, "collecting and owning books" had been his *"favourite hobby"*—if not quite an addiction.[101]

By way of the botanical monograph he had actually written, Freud arrived at the stirring conversation with Dr. Königstein. "Hobby" served as another path to that conversation. The matter they discussed, a matter that never failed to arouse Freud's feelings, was the criticism he had incurred for his absorption in hobbies. At this point he stopped disclosing his associations and provided a mere synopsis of the dream thoughts: they consisted, he claimed, of a "passionately agitated plea" on behalf of his "liberty to act" as he "chose . . . and to govern" his life as "seemed right" to him and to him alone. "After all," he added, "I'm the man who wrote the valuable and memorable paper (on cocaine)."[102]

He stopped short of revealing the struggle he was waging. The dream's manifest content, he noted, with its "indifferent ring," reminded "one of the peace that has descended upon a battlefield strewn with corpses," and for all his indiscretion and audacity, he was loath to identify the dead in public.[103] In his correspondence with Fliess he displayed no such reticence. On January 16, 1898, he vented the full measure of his wrath at Breuer: "I still owe him money from my student days. . . . I succeeded in sending him, with a few words of apology, the first installment." Breuer then made efforts to recompute, downward, the amount outstanding—and Freud was furious: "All this with the greatest lack of logic, with disdainful condescension and deeply hurt feelings, as well as an unabated need to do good. . . . It is genuine Breuer. It is enough to make one extremely ungrateful for good deeds." On January 22 Freud exploded again:

> My anger at Breuer is constantly being refueled. Recently I was disturbed to hear from a patient that mutual acquaintances had said that Breuer severed his relationship with me because he disapproved of the way in which I conduct my life and money matters—a man who earns so much money must save some of it and think of the future. . . . Did he really think I would start saving money *before* I had paid back my old debts for my education?[104]

The conversation with Dr. Königstein had probably refueled Freud's anger once again. Breuer had been a generous friend, if not quite an indulgent father; the relationship had gone sour; now Freud was in a rage at being still in his mentor's debt. Take Breuer away and give him Fliess instead—so Freud had interpreted the wish in his Irma dream. Yet he did not want Fliess to be another Breuer. What did he want?

He did not immediately send his latest daydream and dream interpretation to "the friend whose agreement he recalled with satisfaction." He waited until May 1, 1898.[105] Three weeks earlier the *Wiener klinische Rundschau* had published a highly critical review of Fliess's book: it characterized one passage as "disgusting prattle."[106] Freud, who was a member of the editorial board, demanded a retraction, and when that demand was not met, resigned forthwith. (He also dreamt about the incident.)[107] Only after he had behaved chivalrously toward Fliess, did he send his friend the dream of the botanical monograph—followed by this message: "I am so immensely glad that you are giving me the gift of the Other, a critic and reader—and one of your quality at that. I cannot write entirely without an audience, but do not at all mind writing only for you."[108]

.   .   .

Work on *The Interpretation of Dreams* did not progress smoothly. On October 23, 1898, Freud wrote Fliess: "The dream [book] is lying still, immutably; I lack the incentive to finish it for publication. . . . I am completely lonely."[109] He continued, nonetheless, to record his dreams, among them the following:

I had gone to Brücke's laboratory at night, and, in response to a gentle knock on the door, I opened it to (the late) Professor Fleischl, who came in with a number of strangers and, after exchanging a few words, sat down at his table. This was followed by a second dream. My friend Fl. [Fliess] had come to Vienna unobtrusively in July. I met him in the street in conversation with my (deceased) friend P., and went with him to some place where they sat opposite each other as though they were at a small table. I sat in front at its narrow end. Fl. spoke about his sister and said that in three-quarters of an hour she was dead, and added some such words as "that was the threshold." As P. failed to understand him. Fl. turned to me and asked me how much I had told P. about his affairs. Whereupon, overcome by strange emotions, I tried to explain to Fl. that P. (could not understand anything at all, of course, because he) was not alive. But what I actually said—and I myself noticed the mistake—was, "NON VIXIT." I then gave P. a piercing look. Under my gaze he turned pale; his form grew indistinct and his eyes a

139

sickly blue—and finally he melted away. I was highly delighted at this and I now realized that Ernst Fleischl, too, had been no more than an apparition, a "revenant" [ghost—literally, "one who returns"]; *and it seemed to me quite possible that people of that kind only existed so long as one liked and could be got rid of if someone else wished it.*[110]

A few days before dreaming the dream, Freud noted, he had visited the cloisters of the university for the unveiling of a memorial to Fleischl and had seen again the statue erected in honor of Brücke. During the ceremony, he surmised, he "must have reflected (unconsciously) . . . on the fact that the premature death" of his "brilliant friend P. . . . had robbed him of a well-merited claim to a memorial in these same precincts."[111] (From 1876 to 1882 Freud had worked at the Vienna Physiological Institute; Ernst Brücke [1819–1892] was its chief, and Ernst Fleischl von Marxow [1846–1891] was one of his two assistants. When Freud left, his place was taken by Josef Paneth [1857–1890]). The dating of the dream itself—give or take a couple of days—is thus straightforward: October 30, 1898. The dating of its interpretation is much less so.

Freud recorded his dreams; he did not, however, invariably interpret them or interpret them completely.

> The interpretation of a dream cannot always be accomplished at a single sitting. When we have followed a chain of associations, it not infrequently happens that we feel our capacity exhausted; nothing more is to be learnt from the dream that day. The wisest plan then is to break off and resume our work another day. . . . This procedure might be described as "fractional" dream-interpretation.

Such a procedure, it should become clear, Freud applied to the dream just quoted. He initially interpreted it just after he dreamt it. He returned to it some months later—and, as was true with other dreams he had recorded but whose interpretation he had broken off, the later interpretations complemented the earlier: "When making these subsequent interpretations I have compared the dream-thoughts that I elicited at the time of the dream with the present, usually far more copious, yield, and I have always found that the old ones are included among the new."[112] In the present case both old and new were represented in the dream by the Latin words *non vixit*, which were printed in block letters and gave the dream its name.

That he feared for Fliess's life was the first and immediate interpretation Freud made:

> I had heard from my friend in Berlin . . . that he was about to undergo an operation and that I should get further news of his condition from some of his relatives in Vienna. The first reports I received after the operation were not reassuring and made me feel anxious. I should have preferred to go to him myself but just at that time I was the victim of a painful complaint which made movement of any kind a torture to me.
>
> . . . . .
>
> His only sister . . . had . . . died in early youth after a very brief illness. (In the dream *Fl. spoke about his sister and said that in three-quarters of an hour she was dead.*) I must have imagined that his constitution was not much more resistant than his sister's and that, after getting some much worse news of him, I should make the journey after all—and arrive *too late,* for which I might never cease to reproach myself.

This fantasy, a fantasy that belonged to the dream thoughts, Freud noted, "insistently demanded *'Non vivit'* . . . : 'You have come too late, he is no longer alive.'"[113] Instead *non vixit*—he did not live—had turned up in the dream.

Thoughts of Fliess's death prompted worry about being late; thoughts about his father's death had prompted, the night after the funeral almost exactly two years earlier, a dream with a similar theme. Within days Freud had interpreted and reported it to Fliess:

> I was in a place where I read a sign: You are requested to close the eyes. I immediately recognized the location as the barbershop I visit every day. On the day of the funeral I was kept waiting and therefore arrived a little late at the house of mourning. At that time my family was displeased with me because I had arranged for the funeral to be quiet and simple, which they later agreed was quite justified. They were also somewhat offended by my lateness. The sentence on the sign has a double meaning: one should do one's duty to the dead (an apology as though I had not done it and were in need of leniency), and the actual duty itself. The dream thus stems from the inclination to self-reproach that regularly sets in among the survivors.[114]

Anniversary reactions were no novelty to Freud,[115] and as the end of October approached, he would have been on the alert for representations of his father's death. Once again the dream thoughts would have demanded *non vivit*, not *non vixit*.

Why *non vixit*? Even while dreaming Freud had noticed his mistake, and on awakening he felt obliged to account for it. With some difficulty he remembered that he had seen the words on a statue dedicated to the Emperor Joseph II. And while recalling the inscription, he made yet another mistake: he substituted *patriae*, fatherland, for *publicae*, public.[116] His slip, one he was not aware of until many years later, provides a clue to a chain of dream thoughts he merely hinted at: someone who had lived for the fatherland; someone who owed his life to his father; someone who had not lived. The trail led to Freud's younger brother Julius, who had been born in the autumn of 1857 and had died the following spring just as Freud himself was turning two.[117] Early in his self-analysis he had fathomed the significance of this sibling and had passed along his insight to Fliess: "I greeted my one-year-younger-brother . . . with adverse wishes and genuine childhood jealousy; and . . . his death left the germ of [self-] reproaches in me."[118] Here was a wish. Here was self-reproach—the original self- reproach. Here also the dream thoughts insistently demanded *non vixit*.

Recall that Freud's dream book was "lying still," and his self-analysis presumably lying fallow. Freud himself was "suffering from boils," one of which "the size of an apple had risen at the base" of his "scrotum." "Feverish lassitude, loss of appetite and the hard work with which I nevertheless carried on—all these had combined with the pain to depress me. I was not properly capable of discharging my medical duties."[119] One may speculate that with the intellectual riddle of *non vixit* solved, Freud felt that he had discharged his interpretive duties.

His health improved; his mood brightened; his self-analysis resumed; his dream book perked up. On May 28, 1899, he reported to Fliess that the book was "suddenly taking shape": "This time I am sure of it. I have decided that I cannot use any . . . disguises, nor can I afford to give up anything because I am not rich enough to keep my finest and probably my only lasting discovery to myself." By August 1, he had decided to insert "a small collection of dreams (harmless, absurd dreams; calculations and speeches in dreams; affects in dreams)."[120] By the end of the month that task of incorporation was complete. Sometime, then, during the summer of 1899 Freud subjected the *non vixit* dream to a second interpretive go-round, pressing it into service to illustrate both speeches and affects.

Non vixit had not yet been fully plumbed. Freud fastened on a homonym: the Latin *vixit* and the German *wichsen,* "pronounced like the English 'vixen'" and meaning, "in the language of later childhood," to hit.[121] He associated to a very early scene:

> Two children had a dispute about some object. . . . Each of them claimed to have *got there before the other* and therefore to have a better right to it. They came to blows and might prevailed over right. On the evidence of the dream, I may myself have been aware that I was in the wrong *("I myself noticed the mistake").* However . . . I was the stronger and remained in possession of the field. The vanquished party hurried to his grandfather—my father—and complained about me, and I defended myself in . . . words which I know from my father's account: "I hit him 'cos he hit me."[122]

Dream thoughts about his nephew John, Freud's "inseparable" companion until the age of three and comrade-in-arms in the screen memory of the green meadow and yellow flowers, whom he loved and fought with, insistently demanded the German *wichsen.*[123]

In his paper on screen memories Freud related how he and his nephew had separated: both families had left Freiberg, his migrating to Vienna, John's to Manchester. When he was fourteen, his nephew reappeared, like a revenant. Freud associated to John's visit. The "hitting" resumed: with John taking the part of Caesar and Freud that of Brutus, the two adolescents performed a dialogue from Schiller's play *Die Räuber.* Freud associated to lines from Shakespeare: "As Caesar loved me, I weep for him; as he was fortunate, I rejoice at it; as he was valiant, I honour him; but, as he was ambitious, I slew him."[124]

A year before he dreamt the *non vixit* dream, Freud had written Fliess that his nephew had "determined" what was "neurotic," but also what was "intense," in all his friendships.[125] In associating to the dream, he elaborated:

> All my friends have in a certain sense been reincarnations of the first figure . . . : They have been *revenants.* . . . My emotional life has always insisted that I should have an intimate friend and a hated enemy. I have always been able to provide myself afresh with both, and it has not

143

infrequently happened that the ideal situation of childhood has been so completely reproduced that friend and enemy have come together in a single individual.

Freud further appreciated that thoughts about Fliess's death "could only be construed as meaning" he was "delighted" that it was Fliess, not he, who had died, because, as in the childhood scene, he had been "left in possession of the field."[126] Here he did not elaborate.

On September 21, 1899, Freud sent Fliess galleys of *The Interpretation of Dreams* that included the *non vixit* dream. He drew his friend's attention to the dream and to his pleasure at having outlived him. And then he added, wasn't it "terrible to suggest something" like that?[127] Still he was not deterred. His resolve to use his best material, his own dreams, and to dispense with disguises (his reluctance to reveal sexual content notwithstanding)[128] now allowed him to deliver a stunning message: "It serves you right if you have to make way for me. Why did you try to push *me* out of the way? I don't need you, I can easily find someone else to play with."[129]

.   .   .

One day in the summer of 1901 I remarked to a friend . . . : "These problems of the neuroses are only to be solved if we base ourselves wholly and completely on the assumption of the original bisexuality of the individual." To which he replied: "That's what I told you two and a half years ago at Br. [Breslau] when we went for that evening walk. But you wouldn't hear of it then." It is painful to be requested in this way to surrender one's originality. . . . In the course of the next week I remembered the whole incident, which was just as my friend had tried to recall it to me.[130]

The text is *The Psychopathology of Everyday Life;* the friend, of course, was Fliess; the discussion took place in Achensee in September 1900, not 1901. Freud's forgetting did not happen instantaneously. On March 15, 1898, two and a half months after the Breslau "congress," he wrote Fliess acknowledging bisexuality as a promising field:

I do not in the least underestimate bisexuality . . . I expect it to provide all further enlightenment, especially since the moment in the Breslau marketplace when we found both of us saying the same thing. It is only that at the moment I feel remote from it because, buried in a dark shaft, I see nothing.[131]

A few months later he dreamt about it:

> It [the dream] represented me as laying before my friend [Fliess] a difficult and long-sought theory of bisexuality; and the wish-fulfilling power of the dream was responsible for our regarding this theory (which, incidently, was not given in the dream) as clear and flawless.[132]

In the final, theoretical, chapter of *The Interpretation of Dreams* Freud signaled, albeit in a parenthesis, that he had a stake in the subject.[133] And when he was ready to emerge from the dark shaft of the dream book, he also announced his readiness to enter the lists: "Bisexuality! You are certainly right about it. I am accustoming myself to regarding every sexual act as a process in which four individuals are involved. We have a lot to discuss on this topic."[134] Then there was silence—until the meeting in Achensee. It was the last "congress" the two friends held; it was the last time they saw each other.

The correspondence continued erratically. So too did Freud's pursuit of bisexuality. He mentioned it, he reported to Fliess, in Dora's case history and "specifically recognized" it "once and for all"; he had prepared the ground, he added, "for detailed treatment . . . on another occasion." Before too long he informed Fliess that his next work would be called "Human Bisexuality" and that it would "go to the root of the problem" and would "say the last word" it might "be granted" him to say. (In fact he never did go to the root of the problem: the link between the physiological and the psychical, as always, eluded him, and it was about the psychical, the erotogenic with its multiplicity of meanings, that he chose to have his say.) When Fliess objected, Freud replied: "I do not comprehend your answer concerning bisexuality. It is obviously very difficult to understand each other. I certainly had no intention of doing anything but working on my contribution to the theory of bisexuality."[135] Freud was still determined not to let himself be pushed out of the way—even at the risk of forcing Fliess to make way for him.

By 1902 the correspondence had petered out. Then, in the summer of 1904, Fliess wrote again. He had just come across Otto Weininger's *Geschlecht und Charakter (Sex and Character)*, which had been published the previous year. "In the first . . . part" he had discovered, much to his "consternation," a description of his "ideas on bisexuality and the nature of the sexual attraction consequent upon it—feminine men attract masculine women and vice versa." He had also discovered that Weininger knew Hermann Swoboda, a "pupil" of Freud's, and concluded that it had been from Freud himself, through Swoboda, that Weininger had "obtained knowledge" of his ideas and had "misused someone else's property."[136] Freud initially dodged the issue and then admitted that he had seen a version of Weininger's manuscript before publication: "The underlying theme of bisexuality was of course recognizable, and I must have regretted at the time that via Swoboda . . . I had handed over your idea to him [Weininger]. In conjunction with my own atempt to rob you of your originality, I better understand my behavior toward Weininger."[137] Freud had not succeeded in "mastering the transference in good time."

Conflict within the Transference

> "Up to your *n*th year you regarded yourself as the sole and unlimited possessor of your mother; then came another baby and brought you grave disillusionment. Your mother left you for some time, and even after her reappearance she was never again devoted to you exclusively. Your feelings towards your mother became ambivalent, your father gained a new importance for you," . . . and so on.

Here was a hypothetical example of what Freud called "construction." Was it the case that in laying out such "a piece of early history" before the patient, the analyst behaved according to the principle "heads I win, tails you lose," that is, if the patient agreed, the construction was regarded as correct, and if he disagreed, his disagreement was taken as a sign of resistance, and the construction was still regarded as correct? Not at all, replied Freud. A "plain 'Yes,'" he did not consider unambiguous: it might indicate nothing more than compliance on the part of the patient. A "No" was equally ambiguous: it might actually turn out to be "the expression of a legitimate dissent"—after all, a construction covered "only a small fragment," and dissent might betoken dissatisfaction with its incompleteness. Unless the "direct utterances of the patient" were followed by an indirect confirmation, by the production of new material that completed and extended the construction, those utterances were of no value. In short, Freud concluded, "It will all become clear in the course of future developments."[138]

Recall the case of Ernst Lanzer and the construction Freud had offered him. The process notes make clear what material he had at his disposal: Ernst's adult masturbatory history, a history that began only after his father's death and included oddities, prohibitions, and violations thereof. The published case makes clear what theoretical assumptions Freud was bringing to bear: adolescent or adult masturbation as a revival of childhood masturbation, which itself represented "the discharge of every variety of sexual component and every sort of phantasy" to which such components could "give rise." Though it was only their tenth analytic session, Freud "could not restrain" himself from hypothesizing a specific event: "how before the age of six he [Ernst] had been in the habit of masturbating and how his father had forbidden it, using as a threat the phrase 'it would be the death of you' and perhaps also threatening to cut off his penis."[139]

At the end of the session Ernst allowed that Freud's construction had "brought up a great many ideas in his mind." And at their next meeting he told his analyst what they were:

> The idea of his penis being cut off had tormented him to an extraordinary degree, and this had happened while he was in the thick of studying. The only reason he could think of was that at the time he was suffering from the desire to masturbate. Secondly, and this seemed to him far more important . . . on the occasion of his first copulation . . . [the] idea occurred to him afterwards: "This is a glorious feeling! One might do anything for this—murder one's father, for instance!" This made no sense in his case since his father was already dead.[140]

Finally he narrated the childhood scene, described to him by his mother, of being beaten by his father, being overcome by rage, and hurling epithets such as "You lamp! You towel! You plate!"

Here were "developments" that might stand as indirect confirmation of the analyst's construction. Here were developments which "shook the patient for the first time in his refusal to believe that at some prehistoric period in his childhood he had been seized with fury . . . against the father whom he loved so much."[141] Nonetheless, Freud

147

was disappointed. He felt obliged to admit that he had expected these developments to have had greater effect.

A few years later he would have regarded himself as fortunate that his construction had not disrupted the analysis. In a paper entitled "On Beginning the Treatment" (1913) he warned against proceeding too rapidly:

> It is not difficult for a skilled analyst to read the patient's secret wishes plainly between the lines of his complaints and the story of his illness; but what a measure of self-complacency and thoughtlessness must be possessed by anyone who can, on the shortest acquaintance, inform a stranger . . . that he is attached to his mother by incestuous ties, that he harbors wishes for the death of his wife whom he appears to love, that he conceals an intention of betraying his superior, and so on! . . . Behaviour of this sort . . . will arouse the most violent opposition in him, whether one's guess has been true or not.[142]

.   .   .

At the end of "Fragment of an Analysis" Freud had asked himself whether he might perhaps have kept Dora in treatment if he "had acted a part," if he "had shown a warm personal interest in her—a course which . . . would have been tantamount to providing her with a substitute for the affection she longed for?" He did not know. What he did know was that he had "contented" himself "with practising the humbler arts of psychology." And there were "limits set to the extent to which psychological influence" might "be used," set above all by the "patient's own will and understanding."[143]

More than a decade after Dora had broken off so abruptly, Freud reflected once again on how to avoid such an ending. He had come to appreciate that "psychological influence" could actually foster "the patient's own will and understanding." He had come to appreciate that "the patient's desire for recovery" would induce him to take part in the "joint work," and that "his intelligence" could be assisted by being given "the appropriate anticipatory ideas," that is, by being given some clue as to what was going on.[144] He had come to appreciate that "the first aim of treatment" was "to attach" the patient to it and "to the person of the doctor." He did not recommend playing a part; he did not recommend providing patients with the affection they longed for;

he did, however, recommend "serious interest" and "sympathetic understanding."[145]

In his treatment of Ernst Lanzer Freud put into practice what he was subsequently to preach: he furnished "appropriate anticipatory ideas"; he supplied a sketch of "the underlying principles of psychoanalytic therapy."[146] At the beginning of the fourth analytic session, in response to Freud's query, "And how do you intend to proceed to-day?" Ernst proceeded to tell of his father's death and of how he had come to reproach himself, savagely and obsessively, for having failed to be there at the very end. Here was the opening Freud had been waiting for:

> When there is a *mésalliance,* I began, between an affect and its ideational content (in this instance, between the intensity of the self-reproach and the occasion for it), a layman will say that the affect is too great for the occasion—that it is exaggerated—and that consequently the inference following from the self-reproach (the inference that the patient is a criminal) is false. On the contrary, the [analytic] physician says: "No. The affect is justified. The sense of guilt is not itself open to further criticism. But it belongs to some other content, which is unknown."

At the beginning of the following session, Freud found an occasion to elaborate: "the discovery of the unknown content" ranked as crucial.[147] And to explain why the content should be unknown, he gave Ernst a brief account of the unconscious. He behaved like a teacher telling a student who is looking through a microscope for the first time what he will see; "otherwise he does not see at all, though it is there and visible."[148]

Freud's disquisition did not fully register. Ernst quickly returned to his "natural and spontaneous train of thought."[149] (In his first report of the case for the Wednesday Psychological Society, on November 6, 1907, Freud remarked that he no longer sought "to elicit material" to satisfy his own curiosity, but permitted "the patient to follow his natural and spontaneous trains of thought." If one reads the process notes before reading the paper, one cannot fail to be impressed with the amount of fragmented and confusing material that he was able to keep in mind.)[150] Ernst went on: self-reproach, a "breach of a person's own inner moral principles," and a corresponding "*disintegration of the personality*. . . . Was there a possibility of his effecting a re-integration?" Freud expressed optimism: he "did not dispute the gravity of the case," he told Ernst, but "his youth was very much in his favour." He offered reassurance as well: he ventured "a word or two upon the good opinion" he had "formed of him." This last gave his patient "visible pleasure."[151] Freud was determined to attach Ernst to the treatment and "to the person of the doctor."

In this case Freud's task was no doubt made easier by the fact that he genuinely liked his patient. (Such cannot be said about Dora.) "Serious interest" and "sympathetic understanding" did not require playing a part. At the same time Freud echoed the part played by Ernst's closest friend and confidant, someone he had spoken about during his very first analytic session:

> He had a friend . . . of whom he had an extraordinarily high opinion. He used always to go to him when he was tormented by some criminal impulses and ask him whether he despised him as a criminal. His friend used then to give him moral support by assuring him that he was a man of irreproachable conduct, and had probably been in the habit . . . of taking a dark view of his own life.

It was to this friend that Ernst had turned in his current crisis, a crisis precipitated by hearing of the rat punishment and vowing to repay the wrong person for his new pince-nez.

> When he had arrived in Vienna [from army maneuvers], . . . he . . . had not reached his friend's house till eleven o'clock at night. He told him the whole story that very night. His friend held up his hands in amazement to think that he could still be in doubt whether he was suffering from an obsession, and had calmed him down. . . . Next morning they had gone together . . . to dispatch the 3.80 *kronen* to the post office . . . at which the packet containing the pince-nez had arrived.[152]

Ernst's confidant had had a predecessor, and his natural train of thought during that first analytic session had led him from the former to the latter.

> At an earlier date . . . another person had exercised a similar influence over him. This was a nineteen-year-old student (he himself had been fourteen or fifteen at the time) who had taken a liking to him, and had raised his self-esteem to an extraordinary degree, so that he appeared to himself to be a genius. This student had subsequently become his tutor, and had suddenly altered his behaviour and began treating him as though

he were an idiot. At length he had noticed that the student was interested in one of his sisters, and had realized that he had only taken him up in order to gain admission into the house. This had been the first great blow of his life.

Ernst's opening words, Freud commented in a footnote, thus "laid stress upon the influence over him by men, that is to say, upon the part played in his life by homosexual object-choice."[153] Here were the makings of transference.

In his paper "The Dynamics of Transference" (1912) Freud distinguished a positive and a negative transference. He further subdivided the positive into "friendly or affectionate feelings" that were or were not admissible to consciousness. The feelings that were admissible he regarded as "unobjectionable"—and "the vehicle of success in psychoanalysis" and "in other methods of treatment" as well.[154]

In retrospect Freud ought to have been more suspicious of what seemed "unobjectionable."[155] He ought to have been suspicious of what gained admission to consciousness. He ought to have been on the look-out for unconscious wishes in disguise. In *The Interpretation of Dreams* he had argued that an unconscious wish, to find fulfillment in a dream, transferred its intensity onto a preconscious wish and thereby got itself "covered." The unconscious wish preferred to "weave its connections" around recent and indifferent material in a day's residue.[156] And just as that material served as the point of attachment of a dream wish, so too "some real peculiarity in the physician's person," he noted in "Fragment of an Analysis," served as the point of attachment of unconscious transference wishes.[157] Had he been appropriately suspicious, would he have altered his technique? Would he have attempted to analyze the "unobjectionable" transference? In "Analysis Terminable and Interminable" (1937) he addressed this matter indirectly:

A certain man, who had himself practiced analysis with great success, came to the conclusion that his relations both to men and women—to the men who were his competitors and to the woman he loved—were nevertheless not free from neurotic impediments; and he therefore made himself the subject of analysis by someone else whom he regarded as superior to himself. This critical illumination of his own self had a completely successful result. He married the woman he loved and turned

151

into a friend and teacher of his supposed rivals. Many years passed in this way, during which his relations with his former analyst also remained unclouded. But then, for no assignable external reason, trouble arose. The man who had been analysed became antagonistic to the analyst and reproached him for having failed to give him a complete analysis. The analyst, he said, ought to have known and to have taken into account the fact that a transference-relation can never be purely positive; he should have given attention to the possibilities of a negative transference. The analyst defended himself by saying that, at the time of the analysis, there was no sign of a negative transference. But even if he had failed to observe some very faint signs of it . . . it was still doubtful, he thought, whether he would have had the power to activate the topic . . . by merely pointing it out, so long as it was not currently active in the patient himself at the time. To activate it would certainly have required some unfriendly piece of behaviour in reality on the analyst's part.[158]

In the above case Sándor Ferenczi was the patient and Freud the analyst. In the earlier case of Ernst Lanzer it was the positive transference, not the negative, that remained unanalyzed. The activity of the latter could not have been missed.

.   .   .

On November 30, 1907, Freud noted: "the rat-story becomes more and more a nodal point." Countless "rat-stories . . . disgusting rat-stories," countless permutations and combinations of rat-stories had come tumbling out.[159] There could be no doubt that here was a topic that was currently active—and incomprehensible.

Ernst had begun his narration of the terrible punishment practiced in the East with a sketch of the Czech captain who had told him about it, and of whom he "had a kind of dread." The captain was not a bad man, Ernst reflected, but *"he was obviously fond of cruelty* . . . at the officers' mess he had repeatedly defended the introduction of corporal punishment." And then Ernst had tried to recite the details of the rat punishment—and had failed. Freud had earlier explained to his patient "the idea of 'resistance'": he had given a name to the difficulty Ernst expected to encounter should he attempt "to relate this experience of his." Freud did not interpret the resistance—at least not to his patient. Instead he assured Ernst that he, Freud, "had no taste whatever for cruelty, and certainly had no desire to torment him." But he did precisely that—or so it may well have seemed to Ernst. Freud had made his patient pledge to abide by the fundamental rule of psycho-analysis, and now he refused to release him from that pledge. At the end of the session Ernst "behaved as though he were dazed and bewildered."[160] He had cast Freud in the role of captain, repeatedly addressing him as such.

Recall that in the past Ernst had feared his father, a former noncom-missioned officer and a man with a hasty and violent temper. In the present he feared his analyst: his demeanor on and off the couch—at times, as when attempting to narrate the rat punishment, he would get up and walk about the room—"was that of a man in desperation and one who was trying to save himself from blows of terrific violence; he buried his head in his hands, rushed away, covered his face with his arm."[161]

Here Freud encountered a transference that was not unobjection-able. Here was a transference that had to be mastered in timely fashion if the treatment were to continue. Freud's process notes do not reveal what lines he uttered to accomplish that goal. They do reveal, however, that Ernst plucked up courage and played out a new version of defend-ing his sexual freedom:

> It turned out that he had once met a young girl on the stairs of my house and had on the spot promoted her into being my daughter. She had pleased him, and he pictured to himself that the only reason I was so kind and incredibly patient with him was that I wanted to have him for a son-in-law. At the same time he raised the wealth and position of my family.

On December 8 Freud recorded a dream of Ernst's (Freud did very little with it, or with any other, for that matter): *"He saw my daughter in front of him; she had two patches of dung instead of eyes.* No one who understands the language of dreams will find much difficulty in trans-lating this one: it declared that *he was marrying my daughter not for her 'beaux yeux' but for her money."*[162] Although, Freud wrote after the end of what he regarded as a successful treatment, the "father-com-plex and transference" continued to give his former patient trouble,[163] the father's shadow had been perceptibly lifted from his ego. Ernst remained true to his lady love.

Freud had interpreted Ernst's disjointed narration of the rat punishment as resistance—and had intervened to lessen it. Ernst's countenance had provided further matter for interpretation: "At all the more important moments while he was telling his story his face took on a very strange, composite expression. I could only interpret it as one of *horror at pleasure of his own of which he . . . was unaware.*"[164] To have pointed out his patient's pleasure would certainly have shown "a measure of self-complacency and thoughtlessness." To have pressed Ernst further would certainly have aroused "the most violent opposition." (Here Freud heeded his own subsequent advice: to take care "not to give a patient the . . . translation of a wish" until he was "already so close to it" that he had "only one short step more to make in order to get hold of the explanation for himself.")[165] Instead he simply asked about the identity of the torturer. Ernst replied: "It was not he . . . who was carrying out the punishment, but . . . it was being carried out as it were impersonally"[166]—that is, not by his conscious self. Freud's question had aimed at situating his patient as agent in the narrative.

Only then did he inquire about the person tortured. He guessed that it was Ernst's lady. The surmise was only partially correct. Ernst continued: when the idea had suddenly struck him *"that this was happening to a person who was very dear"* to him, he had immediately deployed "his usual formulas (a 'but' accompanied by a gesture of repudiation, and the phrase 'whatever are you thinking of?')" and had managed to ward off "*both* of them."

> The "both" took me [Freud] aback, and it has no doubt also mystified the reader. For so far we have heard only of one idea—of the rat punishment being carried out upon the lady. He was now obliged to admit that a second idea had occurred to him simultaneously, namely the idea of the punishment also being applied to his father.[167]

What about Ernst's "pleasure"? Rats held the key. In a short interval they had "acquired a series of symbolic meanings," and fresh meanings were continually being added. Those meanings clustered around sexual themes: syphilis—evidently the idea of the disease gnawing and eating had reminded Ernst of rats—this meaning he came to on his own; penis—"itself the carrier of syphilitic infection"—here Freud made the interpretation; worms—Ernst talked about rats gnawing at his anus and then about worms; he had suffered from them, from tapeworms, from large round worms that had moved about in his stool—here Freud set up the equation rat=worm=penis; anal intercourse—the result of a simple substitution, penis for rat—once again Freud took the lead.[168]

What about Ernst as agent? From the outset he located himself as agent in the version of the rat punishment that was being elaborated in the immediacy of the transference. When, during the first interview, Freud told him his fee, he said to himself; "So many florins, so many rats." (Freud learned of this method of payment only a few months later.) Still the payment was being made, as it were, impersonally. That impersonality vanished:

> Things soon reached a point at which, in his dreams, his waking phantasies, and his associations, he began heaping the grossest and filthiest abuse upon me and my family, though in his deliberate actions he never treated me with anything but the greatest respect. His demeanour as he repeated these insults to me was that of a man in despair. "How can a gentleman like you, sir," he used to ask, "let yourself be abused in this way by a low, good-for-nothing fellow like me? You ought to turn me out: that's all I deserve."

Father and lady now merged in the person of the analyst, and Ernst's verbal abuse represented an assault on them both. Was it this re-creation of the rat punishment that Freud had in mind when he wrote, it was "only along the . . . road of transference" that Ernst "was able to reach a conviction" that "he really nourished feelings of rage?"[169]

.   .   .

In the session during which Ernst completed his tale of attempted reimbursement, Freud intervened strictly for purposes of clarification. Here is a part of that tale taken from Freud's published text, which itself represented a clarification of his process notes:

> Argument and counter-arguments had struggled with one another. The chief argument, of course, had been that the premise upon which his vow had been made—that Lieutenant A.[David] had paid the money for him—had proved to be false. However, he had consoled himself with the

thought that the business was not yet finished, as A. would be riding with him next morning part of the way to the railway station at P—, so that he would still have time to ask him the necessary favour [that is, to repay the postal official, and then Ernst in turn would repay A. and thus keep his vow]. As a matter of fact he had not done this, and had allowed A. to go off without him; but he himself had given instructions to his orderly to let A. know that he intended to pay him a visit that afternoon. He himself had reached the station at half-past nine in the morning. He had deposited his luggage there and had seen to various things he had to do in the small town, with the intention of afterwards paying his visit to A. The village in which A. was stationed was about an hour's drive from the town of P—. The railway journey to the place where the post office was . . . would take three hours. He had calculated . . . that the execution of his complicated plan would just leave him time to catch the evening train from P—to Vienna.

Ernst had in fact arrived in Vienna without having accomplished his mission. When he subsequently decided on a new plan—to consult a physician, the choice falling on Freud—he managed to weave that decision into his delusion:

He thought he would get a doctor to give him a certificate to the effect that it was necessary for him, in order to recover his health, to perform some such action as he had planned in connection with Lieutenant A.; and the lieutenant would no doubt let himself be persuaded by the certificate into accepting the 3.80 crowns from him. . . . Many months later when his resistance was at its height, he once more felt a temptation to travel to P—after all, to look up Lieutenant A. and to go through the farce of returning him the money.[170]

A tale, then, of scurrying and scampering that evoked the image of a panicky animal.

Freud did not record how the meaning of Ernst as a rat came to light. He merely provided a summary account:

The notion of a rat is inseparably bound up with the fact that it has sharp teeth with which it gnaws and bites. But rats cannot be sharp-toothed, greedy and dirty with impunity: they are cruelly persecuted and mercilessly put to death by man, as the patient had often observed with horror. He had often pitied the poor creatures. But he himself had been just such a nasty dirty little wretch, who was apt to bite people when he was in a rage, and had been fearfully punished for doing so. He could truly be said to find "a living likeness of himself" in the rat.[171]

Freud did record the following transference fantasy: "My [Freud's] mother's body naked. Two swords sticking into her breast from the side. . . . The lower part of her body and especially her genitals had been entirely eaten up by me and the [other?] children." Freud had interpreted: "The two swords were the Japanese ones of his [patient's earlier] dreams: marriage and copulation. The meaning is clear. . . . Was not the content the idea that a woman's beauty was consumed— eaten up—by sexual intercourse and child-birth."[172] Ernst accepted the interpretation and laughed. He had cast Freud in the role of rat/child. And an oral one to boot.

Analyst and patient alike were discovering the multiple meanings (anal and oral among them) which the erotogenic had bestowed on Ernst and which he was now prepared to transfer to Freud.

.   .   .

Ernst's case, though it was far more satisfactory and satisfying than Dora's, had not entirely opened to Freud's "collection of picklocks." He consoled himself with the reflection that he had been deprived of an opportunity to try out its full range, much wider than it had been in 1900. He had found it impossible, for example, to unravel "thread by thread . . . the tissue of phantasy" in which Ernst's "sexual desires for his mother" and for an older sister and that older sister's premature death "were linked up with the young hero's chastisement at his father's hands." The patient, Freud commented, had recovered: he could now "face life with courage and ability"—father-transference notwithstanding. And that life "began to assert its claims: there were many tasks before him, which he had already neglected far too long, and which were incompatible with a continuation of the treatment." This time it was success rather than failure that accounted for a "gap in the analysis"[173]—mother-transference most conspicuously.

Still, Ernst's case provided sufficient material for Freud to ponder how a "ritual of discourse" might produce "modifications" in the patient. Transference neurosis, a subset of transference phenomena, was the crucial result of Freud's pondering.[174] Transferences or trans-ference reactions, even intense ones, he thought of as displacements of feeling from one object, say, the father, to another, say, the analyst. A transference neurosis he regarded as more organized and systematically elaborated, as an artificial neurosis built around the relationship with the analyst. (Freud's process notes suggest that Ernst's transference, on occasion, fitted this mold.)[175]

> Provided only that the patient shows compliance enough to repect the necessary conditions of the analysis, we regularly succeed in giving all the symptoms of the illness a new transference meaning and in replacing his ordinary neurosis by a "transference-neurosis". . . . It is a piece of real experience, but one which has been made possible by especially favourable conditions, and it is of a provisional nature.[176]

Elsewhere Freud wrote:

> It is not incorrect to say that we [the analysts] are no longer concerned with the patient's earlier illness but with a newly created and transformed neurosis which has taken the former's place. We have followed this new edition of the old disorder from its start, we have observed its origin and growth, and we are especially well able to find our way about in it since, as its object, we are situated at its very centre.[177]

Freud was on the verge of equating the entire therapeutic process with the development of a transference neurosis.

What had happened to remembering? As early as *The Interpretation of Dreams* Freud had expressed his doubts: "the earliest experiences of childhood," he reported having informed a patient, were *"not obtainable any longer as such."*[178] He had pressed screen memories and dreams into service to compensate for childhood amnesia—at a time when he still believed that it was historical reality that he was endeavoring to uncover. And he continued to press them into service when he came to believe that psychical reality—fantasies, some of which might never have been conscious at all and hence not forgotten—was of scarcely less importance. But this was often to no avail. The patient failed to produce a memory of the event or fantasy; instead he produced an action. The patient, it seemed, was obliged "to *repeat*" the unconscious material "as a contemporary experience" rather than "*remembering* it as something belonging to the past." "These reproductions . . . always have as their subject some portion of infantile sexual life—of the Oedipus complex, that is, and its derivatives; and they are invariably acted out in the sphere of the transference, of the patient's relation to the physician."[179] The transference neurosis was a vivid and graphic form of repetition.

Transference itself (and the transference neurosis) now ceased to be an "obstacle"; it became a "powerful ally."[180] It made conflicts accessible to the patient, both affectively and cognitively. As Freud put it, when relics of antiquity, no matter how defined, joined the category of the conscious, they became subject to a process of wearing away. In sketching for Ernst the principles of psychoanalytic theory, Freud had pointed to the antiquities that adorned the room: "They were, in fact, I said, only objects found in a tomb, and their burial had been their preservation: the destruction of Pompeii was only beginning now that it had been dug up."[181] And elsewhere, in a similar vein: "For when all is said and done, it is impossible to destroy anyone *in absentia* or *in effigie*."[182] Or again: "One cannot overcome an enemy who is absent or not within range."[183] Freud had given a new twist to the notion of mastering the transference.

At this point Ernst's question about reintegration became relevant. Freud had taken note of splits in his patient's personality; he had also taken note of projection.[184] He had not quite put the two together: the analyst might represent not only parental figures, or opposing aspects of an ambivalently regarded figure, but a projection of part of the patient's ego—parts of the self that had been cut off from one another and that could not be reintegrated in absentia.

.   .   .

In his *Introductory Lectures on Psycho-Analysis* Freud drew his audience's attention to the fierce objection he was certain his discussion of transference had provoked:

> "Ah! so you've admitted it at last! You work with the help of suggestion, just like the hypnotists! That is what we've thought for a long time. But, if so, why the roundabout road by way of memories of the past, discovering the unconscious, interpreting, and translating back distortions— this immense expenditure of labour, time and money—when the one effective thing is after all only suggestion?"[185]

Freud seized the rhetorical opening he had thus devised. He reminded his listeners that for many years he had practiced hypnotic treatment in combination with prohibitory suggestion. (He might also have reminded them of Janet's treatment of Marie and of how Janet had convinced his patient, while she was in a trance state, that the scene that had figured as traumatic had had, contrary to fact, a happy outcome.) Freud admitted that he had had successes, cases in which the symptoms vanished completely and permanently. He admitted to failures as well, cases in which the symptoms vanished incompletely or not at all. And he did not abandon suggestion entirely. What he wanted to impress upon his listeners was the difference between the prohibitions of hypnotic treatment, designed to "forbid the symptoms," and the *"educative"* purpose of suggestion in psychoanalytic therapy, designed to help the patient overcome resistances to understanding internal conflict.[186]

Hypnosis, Freud had concluded, was not simply unreliable, it was also *"monotonous"* and "hackwork"; it recalled "magic, incantations and hocus-pocus." Above all, it was "not a scientific activity": "in each case, in the same way, with the same ceremonial," the doctor forbade "the most variegated symptoms to exist, without being able to learn anything of their sense and meaning."[187]

Here Freud raised a further objection, once again ascribing it to his audience:

> "If you try to excuse yourself . . . on the ground that you have made a number of important psychological discoveries which are hidden by direct suggestion—what about the certainty of these discoveries now? Are not they the result of suggestion too, of unintentional suggestion? Is it not possible that you are forcing on the patient what you want and what seems to you correct?"[188]

The words echoed those uttered by Fliess more than a decade and a half earlier: "the reader of thoughts" merely read "his own thoughts into other people."[189] After bringing Fliess's criticism into the public arena, Freud was obliged to meet it in order to safeguard his scientific credentials.

He came closest to doing so in his brief remarks about countertransference. In "The Future Prospects of Psycho-Analytic Therapy" (1910), he defined it as the patient's influence on the analyst's unconscious. Two years later he argued that that influence stemmed from the patient's transference. At the same time he seemed to suggest that the concept might cover the analyst's feelings toward the patient in general.[190] (Recall Jones's account of Breuer and Anna O.) This broader scope was implied when Freud warned a younger colleague against "excessive personal interest"; in his own experience, he added, "intensity of feeling" frequently went hand in hand with failure.[191] ("The doctor," Freud wrote, "should be opaque to his patients and, like a mirror, should show them nothing but what is shown to him.")[192] Countertransference, it seemed, frequently went hand in hand with lapses from analytic neutrality as well.[193]

To forestall that danger Freud initially recommended self-analysis and more self-analysis. The analyst should "continually carry it deeper while . . . making his observations on his patients." Anyone, he continued, who failed "to produce results in a self-analysis" should give up the notion of being able to practice psychoanalytic therapy.[194] Given Freud's suspicion—recall his remark to Fliess in 1897 that "true self-analysis" was "impossible"—it was not too long before he revised his recommendation. "Everyone," he insisted in 1912, who wished "to carry out analyses on other people" should himself undergo what soon became known as a training analysis.[195] And that was no easy task—witness Freud's experience with Ferenczi, who was among the first to comply:

> Even a man who is very well able to carry out analyses on other people can behave like any other mortal and be capable of producing the most intense resistances as soon as he himself becomes the object of analytic investigation. When this happens we are once again reminded of the dimension of depth in the mind.[196]

In "Analysis Terminable and Interminable" (1937) Freud sounded an even more somber note. Analysis itself—not simply self-analysis—had, in his view joined the ranks of the "'impossible' professions" in which one could "be sure beforehand of achieving unsatisfying results." (The others were education and government.) Self-analysis, and training analyses as well, came up short. What was to be done? "Every analyst should periodically—at intervals of five years or so—submit himself to analysis once more, without feeling ashamed of taking this step. This would mean, then, that . . . his own analysis would change from a terminable into an interminable task."[197] An interminable analysis stood as Freud's final recommendation to prevent the analyst from reading his own thoughts into his patient's mind.

Along the way he entertained the idea that countertransference itself might be exploited for the purposes of analytic work. He glimpsed something of this possibility when he remarked: "I have . . . good reason for asserting that everyone possesses in his own unconscious an instrument with which he can interpret the utterances of the unconscious in other people."[198] He experienced something of this possibility in his work with Ernst. Recall that the boy's father, in response to his son's fury at being beaten, had declared: "The child will be either a great man or a great criminal!" Freud's father had made a similarly dubious prediction about his small son. The son reported the incident in *The Interpretation of Dreams:*

> When I was seven or eight years old there was . . . [a] domestic scene, which I can remember very clearly. One evening before going to sleep I disregarded the rules which modesty lays down and obeyed the calls of nature in my parents' bedroom while they were present. In the course of his reprimand, my father let fall the words: "The boy will come to nothing." This must have been a frightful blow to my ambition, for references to this scene are still constantly recurring in my dreams and are always linked with an enumeration of my achievements and successes, as though I wanted to say: "You see I *have* come to something."[199]

(The dream of the botanical monograph stood as a case in point.) No wonder Freud was so finely attuned to Ernst's "father-complex."

One is tempted to ask, who is the patient? The analyst himself, Freud insisted, must obey "a counterpart to the 'fundamental rule of psychoanalysis' which is laid down for the patient."

> It consists simply in not directing one's notice to anything in particular and in maintaining the same "evenly-suspended attention" . . . in the face of all that one hears. . . . The rule for the doctor may be expressed: "He should withhold all conscious influences from his capacity to attend, and give himself over completely to his 'unconscious memory'". . . . "He should simply listen, and not bother about whether he is keeping anything in mind."

In short the analyst "must put himself in a position to make use of everything he is told . . . without substituting a censorship of his own for the selection" that the patient has renounced.[200]

In such a position the patient's "ritual of discourse" might produce "modifications" not only in his own person, but in the analyst as well.[201] In no other discipline did the investigator expose himself to so great a risk.

Conclusion:
Let the Exploration Continue

As the twentieth century draws to a close, the controversy over the mind's place—whether mind as well as brain matters—continues to rage. The issue has never been merely philosophical; it has also been one of a research agenda—for or against, as William James put it, accepting as evidence "the feelings of human beings—with heads on their shoulders."[1] Similarly, the divergence between James and Freud over whether to equate the mental or psychical with the conscious—James said yes, Freud said no—went hand in hand with differing research commitments. To take James's line, Freud argued—without mentioning James himself—would force one "to abandon the field of psychological research . . . prematurely," to abandon it "without being able to offer . . . any compensation from other fields."[2] Freud was determined to stick with such research and to explore an unconscious domain construed as mental.

I have charted that exploration along philosophical axes which figured as obstacles—obstacles which Freud was initially loath to confront. He nonetheless did so on the clinical level. He gave a novel twist to traditional problems, and in their new guise they became central concerns of the discipline which was emerging. At this point it may be useful to review the process I have delineated as a series of innovations and applications, and to recall it in words that appeared earlier in the text.

.   .   .

Freud had never been a metaphysician, and he had given up being a physiologist. A philosophical approach to the mind-body problem had thus held little appeal; an experimental approach had been closed off. Despite his marginality—or perhaps because of it—Freud engineered a displacement of the mind-body problem. Preliminaries began when he encountered hysterical patients.

The initial encounter had not been at first hand; it had been with Josef Breuer's patient Anna O. Her symptom of a paralyzed right arm had intrigued Breuer, and after reconstructing its onset, he accounted for it by invoking the notion of conversion, an expression he attributed to Freud. Emmy von N.'s clacking sound, a "succession of sounds which were convulsively emitted and separated by pauses,"[3] Freud considered another example of the same process. Elisabeth von R.'s leg pains proved harder to fit to the mold. Freud could not discern the point at which conversion had taken place in the past. He could discern it taking place in the present: when his patient recalled certain memories and was under the influence of those recollections, she experienced sharp, painful sensations in her legs. The pains had "joined in" the therapeutic conversation. Freud's enthusiasm for conversion, however, did not last; the incomprehensibility of "the leap from a mental process to a somatic innervation" dampened his zeal.[4] Dora's *tussis nervosa* he explained by introducing the concept of somatic compliance: hysterical symptoms, he now argued, involved the participation of both somatic and psychical components. He thereby quietly abandoned his attempt to run a causal sequence from the psyche to the soma, to argue that emotionally charged ideas were converted into somatic symptoms.

Freud may have dreamed of running a causal sequence from the soma to the psyche; he may have wished to discover the solid organic ground for his psychology; but in waking life he was obliged to admit that he could not fit together the organic and the psychological. Paradoxically, his turn to sexuality had the effect of reinforcing his commitment to the psychical. (What other bodily process so readily suggested that a "demand" was being "made upon the mind for work?")[5] Freud's view of sexuality as psychosexual, as a linkage between somatic sexual excitation and psychical sexual ideas—recall that psychic insufficiency figured as the culprit in anxiety neurosis—made possible a crucial step: his conceptualization of the erotogenic. An erotogenic zone was initially bound up with something somatic, with a vital bodily function; subsequently it became separated from bodily needs; it became an archive of experiences of satisfaction. (Those experiences themselves remained conceptually undeveloped.) The body had ceased to be merely physiological.

The application of the notion of erotogenic to the ego marked a further crucial step: "the ego" was "first and foremost a bodily ego."[6] And so it had been in the cases of Little Hans and Daniel Paul Schreber. Even before he had started "setting . . . problems" for his parents, the boy had displayed "a quite peculiarly lively interest in his wiwi-maker." That it played a role in sexual intercourse, his parents never informed him. Yet he had premonitions; he listened, Freud was certain, to the "sensations of his penis." He told his father of thinking something, something forbidden: "I went with you on the train, and we smashed a window and the policeman took us off with him." Father and son had joined forces. Hans also reported a fantasy: *"In the night there was a big giraffe in the room and a crumpled one; and the big one called out because I took the crumpled one away from it. Then it stopped calling out; and then I sat down on top of the crumpled one."*[7] Here father (the big giraffe) and son had a falling out. The boy got his way; he took possession of his mother as crumpled giraffe. Schreber, for his part, claimed that a medical examination would reveal a retreating penis and swelling breasts. But a retreating penis and swelling breasts were only the beginning; it was experiences of sensuous pleasure, particularly when thinking of "something feminine," that served to convince Schreber of his own femininity. He was certain that he was being transformed into a woman, that he would be impregnated by divine rays and give birth to a new race of men.[8] The erotogenic had fashioned Hans's maleness; it could also fashion femaleness, even in a man. It could endow the ego with more than one meaning.

.   .   .

Freud had never been an epistemologist. The philosophical question of how a subject comes to know the object world held no fascination. Archeology was another matter. Freud's adolescent "bibliophile propensities" had given way to archeological propensities;[9] collecting and owning books had been succeeded by collecting and owning antiquities. His being too much absorbed in favorite hobbies was a common criticism leveled at Freud. In this instance, being too much absorbed in archeology made him curiously blind to the displacement of the subject-object problem he had wrought.

The displacement might well have begun when Freud found himself obliged to abandon the seduction hypothesis. In formulating that hypothesis he had invited history, and along with it the object world, into the unconscious domain; in retreating from it, he had no wish to withdraw his invitation. Historical reality might be difficult to uncover; but he was determined to continue his excavation. And so he persisted. He was convinced that screen memories and dreams could undo amnesia about events in childhood—that is, if one knew how to extract those events by analysis. The most dramatic example thereof was Freud's extracting a primal scene from Sergei's dream of six or seven wolves sitting in a tree. In the end Freud's confidence in his analytic work wavered: the scene of observing parental intercourse, he admitted, might not have been part of his patient's personal history; it might have been—indeed it "unquestionably" had been—"an inherited endowment, a phylogenetic heritage."[10] Instead of bracketing the exact relationship between the present and the past, as he had bracketed the exact relationship between the erotogenic and the physiological, Freud invoked phylogenetic inheritance.

The displacement began in earnest when he found himself obliged to contrive a substitute etiology for the abandoned seduction hypothesis. He took the first step when he applied the notion of psychosexuality—a notion that he had first introduced in his work on the actual neuroses—to the defense neuroses as well. Masturbation served as the point of departure. Masturbation, however, as it figured in Dora's case, remained unelaborated. During the next decade Freud expanded its psychical component, construing it as a compound of behavior and fantasy. He had not yet contrived a new etiology.

The work thus far had been merely preparatory. A crucial step came with the application of psychosexuality to love objects. Here oedipal objects emerged. Choosing mother (or her surrogate) over father—the choice Ernst Lanzer hesitated to make—represented a simplification of relationships with two objects toward whom the child felt both love and hate, a simplification with two objects that, Freud claimed, the child's impulses and fantasies had fashioned. (He left the mother undeveloped.) The child, so the argument ran, had soldered together objects and sexually saturated fantasies to produce the Oedipus complex, the nuclear complex of the neuroses.

Freud did still more. He took another crucial step in imagining the "shadow" of an object, soldered together with sexually saturated fantasy, falling on the ego, and the ego itself being altered in the process. He imagined such a process, such a transformation of the subject by the object, occurring only in the wake of the subject's abandoning or relinquishing that object. And so it had been, Freud argued, in Leonardo and Sergei's childhoods. Leonardo had lingered too long over his mother, and in detaching himself from her, a smile, not a shadow, had fallen on his ego. He identifed with her: he put himself in her place, and he loved boys the way she had "loved *him* when he was a child."[11] Sergei had lingered too long over his father; he had renounced his wish to be loved by him only when terrified by what the fulfillment of that wish would entail: castration. The loved and feared object was incorporated into Sergei's ego: from then on ambivalence toward every father-surrogate dominated his being. Leonardo had been "robbed . . . of a part of his masculinity;"[12] Sergei had been blocked on his way to it. In both cases anatomy and destiny had parted company.

·   ·   ·

In displacing traditional philosophical problems, Freud opened up a gap that eventually defined the limits of his enterprise. He had been obliged to abandon whatever hopes he had entertained—hopes is undoubtedly too strong, dreams or fancies would be more apt—of finding physiological grounding. He was similarly obliged—though here he failed to appreciate his obligation—to abandon hopes of finding historical grounding. For reasons internal to his thought, he gave up or should have given up these aspirations. For reasons external to psychoanalysis, such aspirations were bound to be disappointed: a century after Freud's abortive "Project for a Scientific Psychology" (1895), physiology is not yet in a position to offer a mechanistic accounting; and as for phylogenetic inheritance—his surrogate for personal history—even in Freud's lifetime, his younger co-workers chastised him for his stubborn adherence to a variety of evolutionary biology that had been discredited.[13] Willy-nilly, psychoanalysis was on its own.

It was on its own, but it was not merely self-referential. In subsequent generations Freud's hopes for grounding have been transformed into hopes for support from disciplines regarded as neighbors rather than as family members. The issue is not, if it ever was, one of simple reduction. It is a question of how background knowledge from neighboring fields might lend plausibility to or adjudicate among contending psychoanalytic theories; how, for example, knowledge from the neurosciences might help sort out the claims of competing heirs to Freud's notions of a mental apparatus first sketched in the 1890s, or how knowledge from a range of psychological subdisciplines might buttress one or another rival to Freud's developmental theories of libidinal organization and object love.

Psychoanalysis had not become merely self-referential, but it had become a discipline in its own right. It had become autonomous in tandem with the evolution of particular procedures and practices—the most dramatic product of which was transference. "The patient," Freud told a Clark University audience in 1909, directed "towards the physician a degree of affectionate feeling (mingled, often enough, with hostility)" which was "based on no real relation between them" and which—as was shown "by every detail of its emergence"—could only "be traced back to old wishful phantasies."[14] In the analytic setting it became far more intense and preoccupying, thanks to the patient's compliance with the fundamental rule and the analyst's opacity. Transference might be regarded as "artificial"; yet it was "a piece of real experience . . . made possible by especially favourable conditions. . . ."[15] Here was the best chance to make conscious what had been unconscious. Here was complexity of meaning, vivid and graphic.

Psychoanalysis had become autonomous, as I have tried to demonstrate, thanks to Freud's revolutionary restatement of traditional philosophical problems. And thanks to that same process, he had made good his determination to secure space for an unconscious domain in a scientific age.

Abbreviations / Notes
Selected Bibliography / Index

Abbreviations

F/A Letters	*A Psycho-Analytic Dialogue: The Letters of Sigmund Freud and Karl Abraham 1907–1926,* ed. Hilda C. Abraham and Ernst L. Freud, trans. Bernard Marsh and Hilda C. Abraham (New York: Basic Books, 1965)
F/F Letters	*The Complete Letters of Sigmund Freud to Wilhelm Fliess 1887–1904,* trans. and ed. Jeffrey Moussaieff Masson (Cambridge, Mass.: Harvard University Press, 1985)
F/J Letters	*The Freud/Jung Letters: The Correspondence between Sigmund Freud and C. G. Jung,* ed. William McGuire, trans. Ralph Manheim and R. F. C. Hull (Princeton, N.J.: Princeton University Press, 1974)
GW	Sigmund Freud, *Gesammelte Werke, chronologisch geordnet,* ed. Anna Freud, Edward Bibring, Willi Hoffer, Ernst Kris, and Otto Isakower, vols. 1–17 (London: Imago Publishing Co., 1940–1952), vol. 18 (Frankfurt: S. Fischer Verlag, 1968)
IJP	*The International Journal of Psycho-Analysis*
IRP	*The International Review of Psycho-Analysis*
JAPA	*Journal of the American Psychoanalytic Association*
SE	Sigmund Freud, *The Standard Edition of the Complete Psychological Works of Sigmund Freud,* translated under the general editorship of James Strachey (London: Hogarth Press, 1953–1974)

Notes

Introduction

1. Henri F. Ellenberger, *The Discovery of the Unconscious: The History and Evolution of Dynamic Psychiatry* (New York: Basic Books, 1970); Frank J. Sulloway, *Freud, Biologist of the Mind: Beyond the Psychoanalytic Legend* (New York: Basic Books, 1979); John Forrester, *Language and the Origins of Psychoanalysis* (London: Macmillan, 1980); Patricia W. Kitcher, *Freud's Dream: A Complete Interdisciplinary Science of Mind* (Cambridge, Mass.: MIT Press, 1992).
2. Ellenberger, *The Discovery of the Unconscious,* p. 549.

1. Space for Meaning/Intention/Purpose

1. Charles Darwin, *On the Origin of Species* (1859), in *The Works of Charles Darwin,* edited by Paul H. Barrett and R. B. Freeman (London: William Pickering, 1988), 15: 346.
2. See Freud, "An Autobiographical Study" (1925), in *SE* 20: 52. Compare Abram Kardiner, *My Analysis with Freud: Reminiscences* (New York: Norton, 1977), p. 88. For James's reaction to their encounter, see James to Flournoy, September 18, 1909, *The Letters of William James,* ed. Henry James, 2 vols. (Boston: Atlantic Monthly Press, 1920), 2: 327–328. For Freud's trip to the United States, see Saul Rosenzweig, *Freud, Jung, and Hall the King-Maker: The Historic Expedition to America (1909)* (Seattle: Hogrefe and Huber, 1992).
3. William James, "A Plea for Psychology as a 'Natural Science'" (1892), in *The Works of William James: Essays in Psychology,* under the general editorship of Frederick Burkhardt (Cambridge, Mass.: Harvard University Press, 1979–1988), pp. 272, 275.
4. The classic introduction to James's work remains Ralph Barton Perry, *The Thought and Character of William James,* 2 vols. (Boston: Little, Brown:

1935); see also Gerald E. Myers, *William James: His Life and Thought* (New Haven: Yale University Press, 1986). On the questions treated here, see Philip P. Wiener, *Evolution and the Founders of Pragmatism* (Cambridge, Mass.: Harvard University Press, 1949), pp. 97–128; Lorraine J. Daston, "The Theory of Will Versus the Science of Mind," in William R. Woodward and Mitchell G. Ash, eds., *The Problematic Science: Psychology in Nineteenth-Century Thought* (New York: Praeger, 1982), pp. 88–115; William Woodward, introduction to William James, *Essays in Psychology*, pp. xi–xxxix; Robert J. Richards, *Darwin and the Emergence of Evolutionary Theories of Mind and Behavior* (Chicago: University of Chicago Press, 1987), pp. 409–450; Michael G. Johnson and Tracy B. Henley, eds., *Reflections on "The Principles of Psychology": William James After a Century* (Hillsdale, N.J.: Lawrence Erlbaum, 1990).

5. For a detailed account of Pierre Janet's work, see Henri F. Ellenberger, *The Discovery of the Unconscious: The History and Evolution of Dynamic Psychiatry* (New York: Basic Books, 1970), ch. 6. For discussions of the Society of Psychical Research and the work of Frederic W. H. Myers, see Alan Gauld, *The Founders of Psychical Research* (New York: Schocken, 1968); Frank Miller Turner, *Between Science and Religion: The Reaction to Scientific Naturalism in Late Victorian England* (New Haven: Yale University Press, 1974), ch. 5; J. P. Williams, "Psychical Research and Psychiatry in Late Victorian Britain: Trance as Ecstasy or Trance as Insanity," in W. F. Bynum, Roy Porter, and Michael Shepherd, eds., *The Anatomy of Madness: Essays in the History of Psychiatry*, vol. 1, *People and Ideas* (London: Tavistock Publications, 1985), ch. 9; Janet Oppenheim, *The Other World: Spiritualism and Psychical Research in England, 1850–1914* (Cambridge: Cambridge University Press, 1985), chs. 4 and 6.

6. Perry, *William James*, 2: 160.

7. Eugene Taylor, *William James on Exceptional Mental States: The 1896 Lowell Lectures* (New York: Charles Scribner's Sons, 1983), p. 58.

8. William James, "The Hidden Self" (1890), in Burkhardt, ed., *The Works of William James: Essays in Psychology*, pp. 252–253. For a fascinating discussion of late nineteenth-century therapeutic practices in France, see Anne Harrington, "Hysteria, Hypnosis, and the Lure of the Invisible: The Rise of Neo-mesmerism in *fin-de-siècle* French Psychiatry," in Bynum, Porter, and Shepherd, eds., *The Anatomy of Madness*, vol. 3, *The Asylum and Its Psychiatry* (London: Routledge, 1988), pp. 226–246.

9. James, "The Hidden Self," pp. 266–267, and Ellenberger, *The Discovery of the Unconscious*, p. 362.

10. James, "The Hidden Self," p. 267; see also Pierre Janet, *L'Automatisme psychologique* (Paris: Félix Alcan, 1889), pp. 439–440.

11. William James, *The Works of William James: The Principles of Psychology* (Cambridge, Mass.: Harvard University Press, 1981), 1: 369, 370, 371.

12. Ibid., pp. 371, 375.
13. E. W. Stevens, *The Watseka Wonder* (Chicago: Religio-Philosophical Publishing House, 1887), quoted in ibid., p. 375.
14. James, *Principles,* 1: 376.
15. Stevens, *The Watseka Wonder,* quoted in ibid., p. 376.
16. James, *Principles,* 1: 377.
17. Ibid., pp. 207–208, and James, "The Hidden Self," p. 268 (emphasis in the original).
18. F. W. H. Myers, "The Subliminal Consciousness," *Proceedings of the Society for Psychical Research,* 7 (1891–92): 301–302, quoted in Taylor, *Exceptional Mental States,* p. 42. Compare Freud, *The Interpretation of Dreams* (1900), in *SE* 5: 615.
19. William James, *The Works of William James: Manuscript Lectures,* pp. 70–71. See also Taylor, *Exceptional Mental States,* p. 91, and William James, *The Works of William James: The Varieties of Religious Experience,* pp. 189–192, 402–403. For James's acquaintance with Freud's early work, see Nathan J. Hale, Jr., *Freud in America,* vol. 1, *Freud and the Americans: The Beginnings of Psychoanalysis in the United States, 1876–1917* (New York: Oxford University Press, 1971), p. 183.
20. Perry, *William James,* 2: 78.
21. James, *Principles,* 1: 166, 177 (emphasis in the original).
22. James, *Manuscript Lectures,* p. 29.
23. Ibid., pp. 172–173.
24. Freud, "The Unconscious" (1915), in *SE* 14: 167–168. See also Freud: *The Interpretation of Dreams,* pp. 611–613; "A Note on the Unconscious in Psycho-Analysis" (1912), in *SE* 12: 260; *The Ego and the Id* (1923), in *SE* 19: 16*n;* "Some Elementary Lessons in Psycho-Analysis" (1940), in *SE* 23: 283; *An Outline of Psycho-Analysis* (1940), in *SE* 23: 158.
25. Freud, "Some Elementary Lessons in Psycho-Analysis," p. 286.
26. Josef Breuer and Sigmund Freud, *Studies on Hysteria* (1895), in Freud, *SE* 2: 76*n.*
27. Ernest Jones, *The Life and Work of Sigmund Freud,* vol. 2, *Years of Maturity 1901–1919* (New York: Basic Books, 1955), pp. 185, 315; see also Oppenheim, *The Other World,* p. 245. The Society for Psychical Research had previously published a full account of Josef Breuer and Sigmund Freud's "On the Psychical Mechanism of Hysterical Phenomena: Preliminary Communication" (1893).
28. Freud, "A Note on the Unconscious," pp. 260–262.
29. Ibid., p. 263. Freud also postulated a censorship operating between the Pcs. and the Cs.: see Freud, *The Interpretation of Dreams,* pp. 617–618, and Freud, "The Unconscious," pp. 191–192.
30. Richard Wollheim, *Sigmund Freud* (New York: Viking Press, 1971; reprint, Cambridge: Cambridge University Press, 1990), p. 187. I have drawn

heavily on chapter 6 of this book. See Freud, "Five Lectures on Psycho-Analysis" (1911), in *SE* 11: 25–16. See also Patricia S. Herzog, *Conscious and Unconscious: Freud's Dynamic Distinction Reconsidered,* Psychological Issues, Monograph 58 (Madison, Conn.: International Universities Press, 1991).

31. Freud: "Psycho-Analysis and Telepathy" (1941), in *SE* 18: 177–193; "Dreams and Telepathy" (1922), in *SE* 18: 197–220; "Some Additional Notes on Dream-Interpretation as a Whole" (1928), in *SE* 19: 135–138; *New Introductory Lectures on Psycho-Analysis* (1933), in *SE* 22: 31–56.

32. Freud, "A Note on the Unconscious," p. 266.

33. Freud, "The Unconscious," p. 175 (emphasis in the original), and Wollheim, *Freud,* p. 187–188.

34. Freud, "On Beginning the Treatment (Further Recommendations on the Technique of Psycho-Analysis I)" (1913), in *SE* 12: 141.

35. Freud, "The Unconscious," pp. 175–176; see also pp. 180, 189, 191–192.

36. Ibid., pp. 199–201.

37. Ibid., pp. 201–202.

38. See ibid.; see also Freud, *The Ego and the Id,* p. 20, and *An Outline of Psycho-Analysis,* p. 162. For more informal comments on this point, see March 3, 1909, *Minutes of the Vienna Psychoanalytic Society,* ed. Herman Nunberg and Ernst Federn, trans. M. Nunberg, 4 vols. (New York: International Universities Press, 1962–1975) 2: 167, and Freud to Abraham, December 21, 1914, *F/A Letters,* p. 206.

39. Freud, "The Unconscious," p. 195.

40. Freud, *Introductory Lectures on Psycho-Analysis* (1916–1917), in *SE* 15: 61.

41. On repression, see Freud, "Repression" (1915), in *SE* 14: 146–158.

42. On the title page of *The Interpretation of Dreams* Freud used a quotation from Virgil's *Aeneid:* "Flectere si nequeo superos Acheronta movebo"— "If I cannot bend the higher powers, I will move the infernal regions."

43. Freud, *On Aphasia: A Critical Study* (1891), trans. Erwin Stengel (New York: International Universities Press, 1953), pp. 61, 87. Jackson's three-part piece, "On Affections of Speech from Diseases of the Brain" (1878–1880), which Freud drew on, can be found in James Taylor, ed., *Selected Writings of John Hughlings Jackson* (New York: Basic Books, 1958), 2: 155–204. For commentary on Freud's monograph see Erwin Stengel, introduction to Freud's *On Aphasia,* pp. ix–xv, and by the same author, "A Re-evaluation of Freud's Book 'On Aphasia': Its Significance for Psycho-Analysis," *IJP* 35 (1954): 85–89; Charles Davison, review of Freud's *On Aphasia (A Critical Study),* in *The Psychoanalytic Quarterly* 24 (1955): 115–119; Walter Riese, "Freudian Concepts of Brain Function and Brain Disease," *The Journal of Nervous and Mental Diseases* 127 (1958): 287–307; M. M. Otto, "Freud and Aphasia: An Historical Analysis," *American Journal of Psychiatry* 124 (1967): 815–825; Ana-Maria Rizzuto, "A Hy-

pothesis about Freud's Motive for Writing the Monograph 'On Aphasia',"
IRP 16 (1989): 111–117; Ana-Maria Rizzuto, "The Origins of Freud's
Concept of Object Representation ('Objektvorstellung') in His Mono-
graph 'On Aphasia': Its Theoretical and Technical Importance," *IJP* 71
(1990): 241–248. In this discussion, I have drawn on John Forrester,
Language and the Origins of Psychoanalysis (London: Macmillan, 1980),
pp. 14–29; S. P. Fullinwider, "Sigmund Freud, John Hughlings Jackson,
and Speech," *Journal of the History of Ideas* 44 (1983): 151–158; Mark
Solms and Michael Saling, "On Psychoanalysis and Neuroscience: Freud's
Attitude to the Localizationist Tradition," *IJP* 67 (1986): 397–416; Anne
Harrington, *Medicine, Mind, and the Double Brain: A Study in Nineteenth-
Century Thought* (Princeton, N.J.: Princeton University Press, 1987),
pp. 235–247.

44. Freud, *On Aphasia,* p. 73.
45. Freud, *The Interpretation of Dreams,* p. 615.
46. Freud, "Project," p. 366 (emphasis in the original). See also Freud to
Fliess, December 6, 1896, *F/F Letters,* pp. 207–208; Freud, *The Interpretation of Dreams,* pp. 574, 617; Freud, "Formulations on the Two Principles of Mental Functioning" (1911), in *SE* 12: 221.
47. Freud, *The Interpretation of Dreams,* pp. 130, 160, 598; see also ibid.,
p. 566. For informal comment on Anna Freud's dream, see Freud to Fliess,
October 31, 1897, *F/F Letters* p. 276.
48. Freud, *The Interpretation of Dreams,* p. 551; see also Freud, "An Evidential
Dream" (1913), in *SE* 12: 273–274.
49. Freud, *The Interpretation of Dreams,* p. 553 (emphasis in the original).
50. Ibid., p. 553.
51. Ibid., p. 561 (emphasis in the original). The capitalist/entrepreneur metaphor turns up again in Freud, "Fragment of an Analysis of a Case of
Hysteria" (1905), in *SE* 7: 87, and Freud, *Introductory Lectures,* p. 226.
52. Freud, *The Interpretation of Dreams,* pp. 163, 165, 178. A reading of
Freud's marked copy of W. Robert, *Der Traum als Naturnothwendigkeit
erklärt* (Hamburg: Hermann Seippel, 1886) suggests that this book should
receive more attention that it has to date as a source for Freud's emphasis
on recent and indifferent material. See also Edward Timms, "Freud's
Library and His Private Reading," in Edward Timms and Naomi Segal,
eds., *Freud in Exile: Psychoanalysis and Its Vicissitudes* (New Haven: Yale
University Press, 1988), pp. 65–79.
53. Freud, *The Interpretation of Dreams,* pp. 563–564. For a discussion of
day's residues that explicitly extends the concept to a "portion of the latent
dream-thoughts," see Freud, *Introductory Lectures,* p. 226.
54. Freud, *The Interpretation of Dreams,* p. 165; see also Freud, "Remarks
on the Theory and Practice of Dream Interpretation" (1923), in *SE* 19:
109.

55. Freud, "The Handling of Dream Interpretation in Psycho-Analysis" (1911), in *SE* 12: 94.

56. Freud, *Introductory Lectures,* p. 285; see also Freud, "A Difficulty in the Path of Psycho-Analysis" (1917), in *SE* 17: 141.

2. Redefining the Body

1. Freud, *On Aphasia: A Critical Study* (1891), trans. Erwin Stengel (New York: International Universities Press, 1951), p. 55.

2. Freud, "The Unconscious" (1915), in *SE* 14: 168.

3. Robert R. Holt, "Freud's Theory of the Primary Process—Present Status," in Theodore Shapiro, ed., *Psychoanalysis and Contemporary Science: An Annual of Integrative and Interdisciplinary Studies* (New York: International Universities Press, 1977), p. 65. For an excellent discussion of the mind-body problem in Freud's early work, see Barry Silverstein, "Freud's Psychology and Its Organic Foundation: Sexuality and Mind-Body Interactionism," *The Psychoanalytic Review* 72 (1985): 203–228.

4. Freud, *The Ego and the Id* (1923), in *SE* 19: 26.

5. Freud to Martha Bernays, July 13, 1883, *Letters of Sigmund Freud,* ed. Ernst L. Freud, trans. Tania and James Stern (New York: Basic Books, 1960), pp. 40–41.

6. Freud to Martha Bernays, February 2, 1886, ibid., p. 202.

7. Breuer to Fliess, July 5, 1895, reprinted in Albrecht Hirschmüller, *The Life and Work of Josef Breuer: Physiology and Psychoanalysis* (New York: New York University Press, 1989), p. 315. On the relations between Breuer and Freud, see, in addition to Hirschmüller, Siegfried Bernfeld, "Sigmund Freud, M.D. 1882–1885," *IJP* 32 (1951): 204–217; Siegfried Bernfeld and Suzanne Cassirer-Bernfeld, "Freud's First Year in Practice, 1886–1887," *Bulletin of the Menninger Clinic* 16 (1952): 37–49; Ernest Jones, *The Life and Work of Sigmund Freud,* vol. 1, *The Formative Years and the Great Discoveries 1856–1900* (New York: Basic Books, 1953), pp. 221–267; Ernest Jones, "Freud's Early Travels," *IJP* 35 (1954): 81–84; Max Schur, "Some Additional 'Day Residues' of the 'Specimen Dream of Psychoanalysis,'" in R. M. Loewenstein, L. M. Newman, M. Schur, and A. J. Solnit, eds., *Psychoanalysis—A General Psychology: Essays in Honor of Heinz Hartmann* (New York: International Universities Press, 1966), pp. 45–85; Nathan Schlesinger, et al., "The Scientific Styles of Breuer and Freud and the Origins of Psychoanalysis," in John E. Gedo and George H. Pollock, eds., *Freud: The Fusion of Science and Humanism: The Intellectual History of Psychoanalysis,* Psychological Issues, Monographs 34–35 (New York: International Universities Press, 1976), pp. 187–207. See also Freud, "Josef Breuer" (1925), in *SE* 19: 279–280; Paul F. Cranefield, "Josef Breuer's Evaluation of His Contribution to Psycho-Analysis," *IJP* 39

(1958): 319–322; George H. Pollock, "Josef Breuer," in Gedo and Pollock, eds., *Freud: The Fusion of Science and Humanism,* pp. 133–163.

8. Hans-Horst Meyer, "Josef Breuer," *Neue Österreichische Biographie 1815–1918* 5 (1928): 46, quoted in Hirschmüller, *Josef Breuer,* p. 34.

9. Freud, *An Autobiographical Study* (1925), in *SE* 20: 19.

10. See H. F. Ellenberger, "The Story of 'Anna O': A Critical Review with New Data," *Journal of the History of the Behavioral Sciences* 8 (1972): 267–279. In addition to the documents found by Ellenberger, Hirschmüller discovered further material relating to the case and published both sets of documents in an appendix to his *Josef Breuer,* pp. 276–308. For a thorough account of the information available on Bertha Pappenheim, see Lisa Appignanesi and John Forrester, *Freud's Women* (New York: Basic Books, 1992), pp. 72–86.

11. "Case History Compiled by Josef Breuer," in Hirschmüller, *Josef Breuer,* p. 277; see also ibid., pp. 98–101.

12. Josef Breuer and Sigmund Freud, *Studies on Hysteria* (1893–1895), in *SE* 2: 22–23.

13. Ibid., pp. 22, 24 (emphasis in the original).

14. Ibid., p. 42 (emphasis in the original).

15. Ibid., pp. 24, 29.

16. Ibid., pp. 29, 33, 34, 38.

17. Ibid., pp. 38–39.

18. Ibid., pp. 43, 214 (emphasis in the original).

19. Ibid., p. 214*n.*

20. Ibid., p. 206, and Freud, "On the History of the Psycho-Analytic Movement" (1914), in *SE* 14: 9. The first published use of the term appears in Freud, "The Neuro-Psychoses of Defence" (1894), in *SE* 3: 49.

21. Breuer and Freud, *Studies on Hysteria,* p. 86.

22. For the detection of Frau Emmy von N.'s identity and for biographical information about her, as well as the chronology of her treatment, see Ola Andersson to Dr. Kurt R. Eissler, April 16, 1962, Freud Archives/B24, Library of Congress; H. F. Ellenberger, "L'Histoire d'Emmy von N.," *Evolution psychiatrique* 42 (1977): 519–540; Ola Andersson, "A Supplement to Freud's Case of 'Frau Emmy von N.' in Studies on Hysteria 1895," *Scandinavian Psychoanalytic Review* 2 (1979): 5–16; Oskar Wanner, "Die Moser vom 'Charlottenfels,'" *Schweizer Archiv für Neurologie, Neurochirurgie und Psychiatrie* 131 (1982): 55–68.

23. Breuer and Freud, *Studies on Hysteria,* p. 50.

24. Ibid., p. 48.

25. Ibid., pp. 50, 51, 51*n,* 97.

26. Ibid., pp. 49, 96.

27. Ibid., pp. 56–57.

28. Ibid., pp. 80, 94–95.

29. Ibid., p. 80.

30. Ibid., p. 92.

31. Ibid., p. 54 (emphasis in the original).

32. Ibid., pp. 74*n*, 93 (emphasis in the original). For a somewhat different account, see Freud, "A Case of Successful Treatment by Hypnotism with Some Remarks on the Origin of Hysterical Symptoms Through 'Counter-Will'" (1892–1893), in *SE* 1: 124–125.

33. Freud, "A Case of Successful Treatment by Hypnotism," pp. 121–122 (emphasis in the original). On the correspondence between Darwin's idea of antithesis and that of Freud, see Lucille B. Ritvo, *Darwin's Influence on Freud: A Tale of Two Sciences* (New Haven: Yale University Press, 1990), pp. 181–185.

34. Breuer and Freud, *Studies on Hysteria*, p. 92.

35. For Elisabeth von R.'s identity, see Peter Gay, *Freud: A Life for Our Time* (New York: Norton, 1988), p. 72.

36. Breuer and Freud, *Studies on Hysteria*, pp. 139, 145.

37. Ibid., pp. 135–136.

38. Ibid., p. 137.

39. Ibid., pp. 138, 160.

40. Ibid., pp. 140, 144.

41. Ibid., pp. 145–146.

42. Ibid., p. 156.

43. Ibid., pp. 157, 165, 166. See also Freud, "The Neuro-Psychoses of Defence," pp. 47–48.

44. Breuer and Freud, *Studies on Hysteria*, p. 147.

45. Ibid., pp. 142, 147.

46. Ibid., pp. 148, 297. The expression "join in the conversation" recurs in Freud, "From the History of an Infantile Neurosis" (1918), in *SE* 17: 76. The German is "mitzusprechen": see Freud, *Studien über Hysterie*, in *GW* 1: 212, and Freud, "Aus der Geschichte einer infantilen Neurose," in *GW* 12: 107.

47. Freud, "Notes upon a Case of Obsessional Neurosis" (1909), in *SE* 10: 157.

48. Freud, *Inhibitions, Symptoms and Anxiety* (1926), in *SE* 20: 112.

49. Freud, "Sexuality in the Aetiology of the Neuroses" (1898), in *SE* 3: 273–274.

50. Ibid., pp. 267, 268.

51. Freud to Fliess, February 9, 1898, *F/F Letters*, p. 299.

52. Freud to Fliess, September 19, 1901, p. 450.

53. See Frank J. Sulloway, *Freud, Biologist of the Mind: Beyond the Psychoanalytic Legend* (New York: Basic Books, 1979), pp. 135–237. On the intellectual relations between Freud and Fliess, see also Jones, *The Life and Work of Sigmund Freud*, I: 287–318; Ernst Kris, introduction to Freud,

The Origins of Psychoanalysis, Letters to Wilhelm Fliess, Drafts and Notes: 1887–1902, ed. Marie Bonaparte, Anna Freud, and Ernst Kris, trans. Eric Mosbacher and James Strachey (New York: Basic Books, 1954), pp. 3–47; Iago Galdston, "Freud and Romantic Medicine," *Bulletin of the History of Medicine* 30 (1956): 489–507; Max Schur, *Freud: Living and Dying* (New York: International Universities Press, 1972), pp. 63–222. In addition, see Erik Homburger Erikson, "The Dream Specimen of Psychoanalysis," *JAPA* 2 (1954): 5–56, and his "Freud's 'The Origins of Psycho-Analysis,'" *IJP* 36 (1955): 1–15; Schur, "Some Additional 'Day Residues'"; Patrick Mahony, "Friendship and Its Discontents," *Contemporary Psychoanalysis* 15 (1979): 55–109; Alexander Grinstein, *Freud at the Crossroads* (Madison, Conn.: International Universities Press, 1990). For a speculative and tendentious account of the breakup of the friendship, see Peter J. Swales, "Freud, Fliess, and Fratricide: The Role of Fliess in Freud's Conception of Paranoia" (privately printed, 1982).

54. Freud to Abraham, February 13, 1911, *F/A Letters,* p. 100.

55. Kris, "Introduction," p. 4.

56. See Wilhelm Fliess, *Die Beziehungen zwischen Nase und weiblichen Geschlechtsorganen: In ihrer biologischen Bedeutung dargestellt* (Leipzig and Vienna: Franz Deuticke, 1897).

57. Freud, *Beyond the Pleasure Principle* (1920), in *SE* 18: 45. See also Freud: *Three Essays on the Theory of Sexuality* (1905), in *SE* 7: 176–177; "The Disposition to Obsessional Neurosis: A Contribution to the Problem of Choice of Neurosis" (1913), in *SE* 12: 318*n;* and *Introductory Lectures on Psycho-Analysis* (1916–1917), in *SE* 16: 320. For general reflections on the problems periodicity posed for psychoanalysis, see January 29, 1913, *Minutes of the Vienna Psychoanalytic Society,* ed. Herman Nunberg and Ernst Federn, trans. M. Nunberg, 4 vols. (New York: International Universities Press, 1962–1975) 4: 155–156.

58. Wilhelm Fliess, *Der Ablauf des Lebens: Grundlegung zur exakten Biologie* (Leipzig and Vienna: Franz Deuticke, 1906), quoted in Kris, "Introduction," p. 7

59. Freud, *Beyond the Pleasure Principle,* p. 45.

60. Freud to Fliess, June 30, 1896, *F/F Letters,* p. 193; December 4, 1896, p. 204; December 17, 1896, p. 215; and September 22, 1898, p. 326. See also Freud to Jung, April 19, 1908, *F/J Letters,* pp. 140–141, and November 30, 1911, p. 469.

61. See Sulloway, *Freud: Biologist of the Mind,* p. 171.

62. Freud, "Instincts and Their Vicissitudes" (1915), in *SE* 14: 122.

63. Breuer and Freud, *Studies on Hysteria,* pp. 86, 87.

64. Freud, "On the Grounds for Detaching a Particular Syndrome from Neurasthenia Under the Description 'Anxiety Neurosis'" (1895), in *SE* 3: 96.

65. Breuer and Freud, *Studies on Hysteria,* pp. 74, 74*n*.

66. Freud, "On the Grounds for Detaching . . . 'Anxiety Neurosis,'" p. 96, and Breuer and Freud, *Studies on Hysteria*, p. 88.

67. Freud, "Draft E. How Anxiety Originates" (undated; ?June 6, 1894), in *F/F Letters*, p. 79; see also his "Draft C. Something of a Report on Motives" (undated; ?April 1893), in ibid., pp. 45–47.

68. Freud, "Draft E," p. 79.

69. Freud, "On the Grounds for Detaching . . . 'Anxiety Neurosis,'" pp. 99–100 (emphasis in the original).

70. Freud, "Draft E," p. 79 (emphasis in the original).

71. Freud, "On the Grounds for Detaching . . . 'Anxiety Neurosis,'" p. 101 (emphasis in the original).

72. Ibid. (emphasis in the original).

73. Freud, "Draft E," p. 79 (emphasis in the original).

74. Freud to Fliess, November 27, 1893, *F/F Letters*, p. 61.

75. Freud, "Draft F. Collection III" (August 18, 1894), in *F/F Letters*, pp. 90–91.

76. Freud to Fliess, August 23, 1894, *F/F Letters*, pp. 92–93 (emphasis in the original).

77. Ibid., p. 92.

78. Freud, "Draft E," pp. 79–80 (emphasis in the original).

79. Freud, "On the Grounds for Detaching . . . 'Anxiety Neurosis,'" p. 108 (emphasis in the original); see also his "Draft G. Melancholia" (undated), in *F/F Letters*, pp. 98–105. See also James Strachey, editor's introduction to Freud, "Instincts and Their Vicissitudes," pp. 112–113. For an excellent discussion of Freud's views on sexuality and the actual neuroses, see Walter A. Stewart, *Psychoanalysis: The First Ten Years 1888–1898* (New York: Macmillan, 1967), pp. 42–73.

80. Freud, "On the Grounds for Detaching . . . 'Anxiety Neurosis,'" p. 109. For Freud's later qualification of this theory of the sexual process, see his *Three Essays*, pp. 213–214.

81. Freud to Fliess, August 23, 1894, *F/F Letters*, p. 93 (emphasis in the original).

82. Freud to Fliess, November 27, 1893, p. 61. For the discussion of this case, I have drawn on Stewart, *Psychoanalysis: The First Ten Years*, pp. 55–56.

83. For biographical information about Katharina, see Peter J. Swales, "Freud, Katharina, and the First 'Wild Analysis,'" in Paul E. Stepansky, ed., *Freud Appraisals and Reappraisals: Contributions to Freud Studies* (Hillsdale, N.J.: Analytic Press, 1988) 3: 81–163.

84. Breuer and Freud, *Studies on Hysteria*, p. 260.

85. Ibid., pp. 131.

86. Ibid., p. 133.

87. Freud, "On the Grounds for Detaching . . . 'Anxiety Neurosis,'" p. 110.

88. Ibid., p. 109.

89. Ibid., p. 115 (emphasis in the original).

90. Compare Freud, *Inhibition, Symptoms and Anxiety,* p. 109.

91. Breuer and Freud, *Studies on Hysteria,* p. 137.

92. Freud, "Hysteria" (1888), in *SE* 1: 43.

93. Breuer and Freud, *Studies on Hysteria,* pp. 148, 175.

94. Freud to Fliess, December 6, 1896, *F/F Letters,* p. 212, and November 14, 1897, p. 279. See also Freud to Fliess, January 12, 1897, p. 223.

95. Freud, *Three Essays,* p. 182.

96. Ibid., p. 182.

97. Freud, "Fragment of an Analysis of a Case of Hysteria" (1905), in *SE* 7: 19, 20. For biographical information about Dora, see Hannah S. Decker, *Freud, Dora, and Vienna 1900* (New York: Free Press, 1991). See also "Biographical Note: Dora's Family," in Charles Bernheimer and Claire Kahane, eds., *In Dora's Case: Freud—Hysteria—Feminism* (New York: Columbia University Press, 1985), pp. 33–34, and Felix Deutsch, "A Footnote to Freud's 'Fragment of an Analysis of a Case of Hysteria,'" in ibid., pp. 35–43.

98. Freud, "Fragment of an Analysis," pp. 25, 28, 34, 35.

99. Freud to Fliess, October 14, 1900, *F/F Letters,* p. 427.

100. Freud, "Fragment of an Analysis," pp. 11, 12, 24.

101. Freud to Fliess, January 25, 1901, *F/F Letters,* p. 433, and January 30, 1901, p. 434.

102. Freud, "Fragment of an Analysis," p. 22.

103. Ibid., pp. 22, 40–41, 54, 83.

104. Ibid., pp. 51. For a suggestive discussion of the erotogenic body, see Monique David-Ménard, *Hysteria from Freud to Lacan: Body and Language in Psychoanalysis,* trans. Catherine Porter (Ithaca, N.Y.: Cornell University Press, 1989), pp. 64–104.

105. For a third, fragmentary interpretation, see Freud, "Fragment of an Analysis," p. 82. For a further reference to this interpretation, see Freud, *Group Psychology and the Analysis of the Ego* (1921), in *SE* 18: 106–107.

106. Freud, "Fragment of an Analysis," pp. 59–63, 110*n.*

107. Ibid., pp. 39, 40 (emphasis in the original).

108. Ibid., pp. 46, 47, 48 (emphasis in the original).

109. Freud, "Disposition to Obsessional Neurosis," p. 319. Freud introduced the classification of anxiety hysteria to denote erotic longing transformed into anxiety by the defensive process he had earlier attributed to conversion hysteria: see Freud, "Analysis of a Phobia in a Five-Year-Old Boy" (1909), in *SE* 10: 25–26, 114–115. For his subsequent dissatisfaction with his original formulation, see Freud, *Inhibitions, Symptoms and Anxiety,* pp. 108–109.

110. Freud, "Disposition to Obsessional Neurosis," p. 320.

111. Freud, "The Infantile Genital Organization (An Interpolation into the Theory of Sexuality)" (1923), in *SE* 19: 141–145.

112. Freud, *New Introductory Lectures on Psycho-Analysis* (1933), in *SE* 22: 100.

113. See Freud to Fliess, November 14, 1899, *F/F Letters,* p. 280.

114. Freud, "The Infantile Genital Organization," p. 145 (emphasis in the original).

115. Freud, "Analysis of a Phobia," p. 6.

116. Ibid., pp. 6, 7, 10, 22, 142.

117. Ibid., pp. 24, 124 (emphasis in the original).

118. Ibid., pp. 47, 101, 124. For the notion of a disease plucking up courage, see also Freud, "Notes upon a Case of Obsessional Neurosis," p. 223. Freud used material from the case of Little Hans in two other, related papers: "The Sexual Enlightenment of Children (An Open Letter to Dr. M. Fürst)" (1907), in *SE* 9: 131–139, and "On the Sexual Theories of Children" (1908), in *SE* 9: 207–226. For further discussion of this material, see May 12, 1909, *Minutes of the Vienna Psychoanalytic Society* 2: 227–236. See also Max Graf, "Reminiscence of Professor Freud," *The Psychoanalytic Quarterly* 11 (1942): 465–476.

119. Freud, "Analysis of a Phobia," pp. 7, 9, 13, 14. Strachey translated "Wiwimacher" as "widdler."

120. Ibid., p. 145.

121. Ibid., pp. 40, 41, 122, 135.

122. Ibid., pp. 37, 39, 41 (emphasis in the original).

123. Ibid., pp. 42, 123.

124. Ibid., pp. 34, 35, 36.

125. Ibid., pp. 98, 100.

126. Ibid., pp. 65, 98, 128.

127. Ibid., pp. 105, 127, 128.

128. Ibid., pp. 87, 130.

129. Ibid., pp. 93*n*, 95, 97, 133.

130. Daniel Paul Schreber, *Memoirs of My Nervous Illness,* trans. and ed. by Ida Macalpine and Richard A. Hunter (Cambridge, Mass.: Harvard University Press, 1988), p. 132*n*.

131. Ibid., p. 63. For biographical information on Schreber, see Franz Baumeyer, "The Schreber Case," *IJP* 37 (1956): 61–74; William G. Niederland, *The Schreber Case: Psychoanalytic Profile of a Paranoid Personality* (New York: Quadrangle/New York Times, 1974); Han Israëls, *Schreber: Father and Son,* trans. H. S. Lake (Madison, Conn.: International Universities Press, 1989).

132. Dr. Weber, "Asylum and District Medical Officer's Report" (November 28, 1900), in Schreber, *Memoirs,* p. 278.

133. Dr. Weber, "Medical Expert's Report to the Court" (December 9, 1899), in ibid., pp. 267, 268, 269, 270, 271.

134. Schreber, *Memoirs,* pp. 31, 155*n*, 159.

135. "Judgment of the Royal Superior Country Court Dresden of 14th July 1902," in ibid., p. 354.

136. Daniel Paul Schreber, "Grounds for Appeal" (July 23, 1901), in ibid., p. 307.

137. Freud to Jung, April 22, 1910, *F/J Letters,* p. 311, and December 18, 1910, pp. 379–380.

138. See Freud, "Draft H. Paranoia" (enclosed with letter of January 24, 1895), in *F/F Letters,* pp. 107–112; Freud, "Draft K. The Neuroses of Defense (A Christmas Fairy Tale)" (enclosed with letter of January 1, 1896), in ibid., pp. 167–168; Freud "Further Remarks on the Neuro-Psychoses of Defence" (1896), in *SE* 3: 174–185.

139. Freud to Fliess, December 9, 1899, *F/F Letters,* p. 390.

140. See Freud to Ferenczi, February 11, 1908, and March 25, 1908; Freud to Jung, February 18, 1908, *F/J Letters,* p. 121; Freud, "Psycho-Analytic Notes on an Autobiographical Account of a Case of Paranoia (Dementia Paranoides)" (1911), in *SE* 12: 59–78. See also Sándor Ferenczi, "On the Part Played by Homosexuality in the Pathogenesis of Paranoia" (1912), in his *First Contributions to Psycho-Analysis,* authorized trans. by Ernest Jones (London: Maresfield Reprints, 1980), pp. 154–184.

141. Freud, *Three Essays,* p. 219*n,* and his "The Psychogenesis of a Case of Homosexuality in a Woman" (1920), in *SE* 18: 170–171.

142. Freud, "Psycho-Analytic Notes on . . . a Case of Paranoia," p. 18.

143. Daniel Paul Schreber, *Denkwürdigkeiten eines Nervenkranken,* (Leipzig: Oswald Mutze, 1903), pp. 56, 59, quoted in Freud, "Psycho-Analytic Notes on . . . a Case of Paranoia," p. 19.

144. Ibid., p. 19 (emphasis in the original).

145. Ibid., p. 20.

146. Schreber, *Memoirs,* p. 43*n* (emphasis in the original).

147. Ibid., p. 132 (emphasis in the original).

148. Ibid., p. 207 (emphasis in the original).

149. Ibid., pp. 204, 205 (emphasis in the original).

150. Freud, *Three Essays,* p. 184.

151. Schreber, *Memoirs,* pp. 149, 212.

152. For Freud's use of Napoleon's epigram "Anatomy is Destiny," see Freud, "On the Universal Tendency to Debasement in the Sphere of Love (Contributions to the Psychology of Love II)" (1912), in *SE* 11: 189, and Freud, "The Dissolution of the Oedipus Complex" (1924), in *SE* 19: 178.

3. Redefining the Object

1. Freud to Silberstein, November 8, 1874, *The Letters of Sigmund Freud to Eduard Silberstein 1871–1881,* ed. Walter Boehlich, trans. Arnold J. Pomerans (Cambridge, Mass.: Harvard University Press, 1990), p. 70, and Freud to Silberstein, March 15, 1875, ibid., p. 102. For Freud's encounter

with Brentano, see William J. McGrath, *Freud's Discovery of Psychoanalysis: The Politics of Hysteria* (Ithaca, N.Y.: Cornell University Press, 1986), ch. 3. See also James R. Barclay, "Franz Brentano and Sigmund Freud," *Journal of Existentialism* 5 (1964): 1–36; Raymond E. Francher, "Brentano's *Psychology from an Empirical Standpoint* and Freud's Early Metapsychology," *Journal of the History of the Behavioral Sciences* 13 (1977): 207–227; Patricia Herzog, "The Myth of Freud as Anti-Philosopher," in Paul E. Stepansky, ed., *Freud Appraisals and Reappraisals: Contributions of Freud Studies* (Hillsdale, N.J.: Analytic Press, 1988) 2: 163–189; Michael F. Frampton, "Considerations on the Role of Brentano's Concept of Intentionality in Freud's Repudiation of the Seduction Theory," *IRP* 18 (1991): 27–36; John E. Toews, "Historicizing Psychoanalysis: Freud in His Time and for Our Time," *The Journal of Modern History* 63 (1991): 504–545.

2. Freud to Silberstein, March 15, 1875, *Letters of Freud to Silberstein,* pp. 103, 104.

3. Freud to Silberstein, March 13, 1875, ibid., p. 101, and September 9, 1875, p. 128.

4. Freud to Fliess, January 1, 1896, *F/F Letters,* p. 159, and February 1, 1900, p. 398.

5. Freud, "On the History of the Psycho-Analytic Movement" (1914), in *SE* 14: 15. See also Freud to Putnam, March 30, 1914, *James Jackson Putnam and Psychoanalysis: Letters between Putnam and Sigmund Freud, Ernest Jones, William James, Sándor Ferenczi, and Morton Prince, 1877–1917,* ed. Nathan G. Hale, Jr. (Cambridge, Mass.: Harvard University Press, 1971), p. 170, and Freud, "An Autobiographical Study" (1925), in *SE* 20: 59–60.

6. Freud to Fliess, February 1, 1900, *F/F Letters,* p. 398.

7. See, for example, Freud, "Instincts and Their Vicissitudes" (1915), in *SE* 14: 134.

8. See Freud, *The Ego and the Id* (1923), in *SE* 19: 29–30.

9. See Siegfried Bernfeld, "An Unknown Autobiographical Fragment by Freud," *American Imago* 4 (1946): 3–19.

10. Freud, "Screen Memories" (1899), in *SE* 3: 311.

11. Ibid., pp. 312, 313. I have followed Freud's version in "Screen Memories." In describing both occasions he made himself a year older than he actually was. For his visit to Moravia and his encounter with Gisela Fluss, see Freud to Silberstein, August 17, 1872, *Letters of Freud to Silberstein,* pp. 11–12, and September 14, 1872, pp. 16–19.

12. Freud, "Screen Memories," p. 314. For Freud's trip to Manchester, see Freud to Silberstein, August 3, 1875, *Letters of Freud to Silberstein,* pp. 123–124, and September 9, 1875, pp. 125–128.

13. Freud, "Screen Memories," pp. 312, 314, 315. For a provocative hypothe-

sis about when the memory emerged, see Peter J. Swales, "Freud, Martha Bernays, and the Language of Flowers" (privately printed, 1983).

14. Freud, *Introductory Lectures on Psycho-Analysis* (1916–1917), in *SE* 16: 367.
15. Freud, "Screen Memories," p. 315.
16. Ibid., pp. 316, 320.
17. Ibid., p. 316.
18. Freud, "Remembering, Repeating and Working-Through (Further Recommendations on the Technique of Psycho-Analysis II)" (1914), in *SE* 12: 148 (emphasis in the original).
19. Freud, *The Interpretation of Dreams* (1900), in *SE* 4: 15–16.
20. Ibid., pp. 16–17; see also p. 189.
21. Ibid., p. 17. For a somewhat different account, see Freud *Introductory Lectures on Psycho-Analysis,* p. 201.
22. Freud to Fliess, October 15, 1897, *F/F Letters,* p. 271.
23. For references to the accident, see Freud, "Screen Memories," p. 310, and *The Interpretation of Dreams,* p. 560.
24. Freud, *The Interpretation of Dreams,* p. 275.
25. Freud to Fliess, December 3, 1897, *F/F Letters,* p. 285.
26. Freud, *The Interpretation of Dreams,* p. 195.
27. Freud to Fliess, December 3, 1897, *F/F Letters,* p. 284, and Freud, *The Interpretation of Dreams,* p. 196.
28. For the discussion of this dream, I have drawn on Didier Anzieu, *Freud's Self-Analysis,* trans. Peter Graham (London: Hogarth Press, 1986), pp. 195–213; see also Alexander Grinstein, *On Sigmund Freud's Dreams* (Detroit, Mich.: Wayne State University Press, 1968), pp. 69–91.
29. Freud, *The Interpretation of Dreams,* pp. 197.
30. Ibid., pp. 196, 197. On Freud's fascination with Hannibal, see McGrath, *Freud's Discovery of Psychoanalysis,* pp. 62–66.
31. Freud, *The Psychopathology of Everyday Life* (1901), in *SE* 6: 218 (emphasis in the original). See also Freud to Fliess, November 12, 1899, *F/F Letters,* p. 385.
32. Freud, *Introductory Lectures on Psycho-Analysis,* p. 66.
33. Freud, *The Psychopathology of Everyday Life,* pp. 219–220.
34. Freud, *The Interpretation of Dreams,* pp. 189, 199.
35. Freud, *Introductory Lectures on Psycho-Analysis,* p. 367.
36. Freud, "Constructions in Analysis" (1937), in *SE* 23: 267 (emphasis in the original).
37. Freud, *Moses and Monotheism: Three Essays* (1939), in *SE* 23: 130.
38. See Freud, "Further Remarks on the Neuro-Psychoses of Defence" (1896), in *SE* 3: 184; Freud, *The Psychopathology of Everyday Life,* p. 256; Freud, "Delusions and Dreams in Jensen's *Gradiva*" (1907), in *SE* 9: 80;

Freud, "Some Neurotic Mechanisms in Jealousy, Paranoia and Homosexuality" (1922), in *SE* 18: 226.

39. Freud, "Fragment of an Analysis of a Case of Hysteria" (1905), in *SE* 7: 12. See also Josef Breuer and Sigmund Freud, *Studies on Hysteria* (1893–1895), in *SE* 2: 139; and Freud: "The Aetiology of Hysteria" (1896), in *SE* 3: 192; "Jensen's *Gradiva*," p. 40; "Notes upon a Case of Obsessional Neurosis" (1909), in *SE* 10: 177; and "Constructions in Analysis," pp. 259–260.

40. "My Recollections of Sigmund Freud," in Muriel Gardiner, ed., *The Wolf-Man by the Wolf-Man* (New York: Basic Books, 1971), p. 139. See also Suzanne Cassirer Bernfeld, "Freud and Archaeology," *American Imago* 8 (1951): 107–128.

41. Freud, "Jensen's *Gradiva*," pp. 8, 41.

42. Ibid., p. 14.

43. Ibid., p. 10.

44. Wilhelm Jensen, *Gradiva: Ein pompejanisches Phantasiestück* (Dresden and Leipzig: Carl Reissner, 1903), p. 4. The copy I have used is Freud's own (with his marginal comments), which is in the Freud Museum, London.

45. Freud, "Jensen's *Gradiva*," p. 12.

46. Jensen, *Gradiva*, p. 2.

47. Freud, "Jensen's *Gradiva*," pp. 12–13.

48. Ibid., p. 13.

49. Jensen, *Gradiva*, p. 24.

50. Freud, "Jensen's *Gradiva*," p. 15.

51. Jensen, *Gradiva*, p. 58.

52. Ibid., p. 69.

53. Freud, "Jensen's *Gradiva*," pp. 18, 19.

54. Jensen, *Gradiva*, p. 69.

55. Freud, "Jensen's *Gradiva*," pp. 20, 21.

56. Jensen, *Gradiva*, p. 120.

57. Freud, "Jensen's *Gradiva*," p.30.

58. Jensen, *Gradiva*, pp. 136, 138.

59. Freud, "Jensen's *Gradiva*," pp. 31, 36, 37.

60. Jensen, *Gradiva*, p. 142.

61. Freud, "Jensen's *Gradiva*," pp. 31, 37. Freud was curious about Jensen's own opinion and wrote him a letter of inquiry. For the subsequent correspondence, see Freud to Jung, May 26, 1907, *F/J Letters,* p. 52; November 24, 1907, p. 100, and December 21, 1907, pp. 104–105; see also "Drei unveröffentlichte Briefe von Wilhelm Jensen," *Psychoanalytische Bewegung* 1 (1929): 207–211. See also November 20, 1907, *Minutes of the Vienna Psychoanalytic Society,* ed. Herman Nunberg and Ernst Federn, trans. M. Nunberg, 4 vols. (New York: International Universities Press, 1962–1975) 1: 246–247.

62. Freud to Fliess, September 21, 1897, *F/F Letters,* p. 264 (emphasis in the original).
63. See Freud, "Further Remarks on the Neuro-Psychoses of Defence," pp. 162–185; see also Freud: "Draft K. The Neuroses of Defense (A Christmas Fairy Tale)" (enclosed with letter of January 1, 1896), in *F/F Letters,* pp. 162–169; "Heredity and the Aetiology of the Neuroses" (1896), in *SE* 3: 151–156; and "The Aetiology of Hysteria," pp. 199–221.
64. Freud to Fliess, September 21, 1897, *F/F Letters,* p. 265. Compare Freud, "Further Remarks on the Neuro-Psychoses of Defence," p. 164*n,* and Freud to Fliess, December 12, 1897, *F/F Letters,* p. 286. See also Freud: "My Views on the Part Played by Sexuality in the Aetiology of the Neuroses" (1906), in *SE* 7: 274–275; "History of the Psycho-Analytic Movement," pp. 17–18; and "An Autobiographical Study," pp. 34–35. Why Freud abandoned the seduction hypothesis has been much debated: see in particular, Ernest Jones, *The Life and Work of Sigmund Freud,* vol. 1, *The Formative Years and the Great Discoveries 1866–1900* (New York: Basic Books, 1953), pp. 263–267; Kenneth Levin, *Freud's Early Psychology of the Neuroses: A Historical Perspective* (Pittsburgh, Pa.: University of Pittsburgh Press, 1978); Marie Balmary, *Psychoanalyzing Psychoanalysis: Freud and the Hidden Fault of the Father,* trans. Ned Lukacher (Baltimore: Johns Hopkins University Press, 1982); Peter J. Swales, "Freud, Johann Weier, and the Status of Seduction: The Role of the Witch in the Conception of Fantasy" (privately printed, 1982); Peter J. Swales, "Freud, Krafft-Ebing, and the Witches: the Role of Krafft-Ebing in Freud's Flight into Fantasy" (privately printed, 1983); Jeffrey Moussaieff Masson, *The Assault on Truth: Freud's Suppression of the Seduction Theory* (New York: Farrar, Straus and Giroux, 1984); Marianne Krüll, *Freud and His Father,* trans. Arnold J. Pomerans (New York: Norton, 1986). For a masterly critique of Masson, see Paul Robinson, *Freud and His Critics* (Berkeley: University of California Press, 1993).
65. Though Freud retracted his assertion that at the root of *every* hysteria lay a passive sexual experience, namely seduction, he did not deprive seduction of a role in *some* hysterias. See Freud, "Further Remarks on the Neuro-Psychoses of Defence," p. 168*n;* Breuer and Freud, *Studies on Hysteria,* p. 134*n;* Freud: *Introductory Lectures on Psycho-Analysis* p. 370; "Female Sexuality" (1931), in *SE* 21: 232; and *An Outline of Psycho-Analysis* (1940), in *SE* 23: 187.
66. Freud, "Fragment of an Analysis of a Case of Hysteria" (1905), in *SE* 7: 11.
67. Ibid., p. 64.
68. Freud, *The Interpretation of Dreams,* p. 190.
69. Freud, "Fragment of an Analysis," p. 64 (emphasis in the original).
70. Ibid., pp. 64, 65.

71. Freud, "History of the Psycho-Analytic Movement," p. 10.
72. Freud, "Fragment of an Analysis," p. 69.
73. Ibid., pp. 65, 72 (emphasis in the original).
74. Freud, *Three Essays on the Theory of Sexuality* (1905), in *SE* 7: 190.
75. Freud, "Fragment of an Analysis," pp. 75, 76.
76. See ibid., pp. 79, 79*n*.
77. Freud, "History of the Psycho-Analytic Movement," p. 17 (emphasis in the original).
78. In April 1908 the Wednesday Psychological Society changed to the more formal title of Vienna Psychoanalytic Society.
79. January 24, 1912, *Minutes of the Vienna Psychoanalytic Society* 4: 24–25; see also Freud, *New Introductory Lectures on Psycho-Analysis* (1933), in *SE* 22: 120.
80. Freud, "Hysterical Phantasies and Their Relation to Bisexuality" (1908), in *SE* 9: 161, and Freud, "Hysterische Phantasien und Ihre Beziehung zur Bisexualität," in *GW* 7: 193.
81. Freud to Fliess, July 7, 1897, *F/F Letters*, p. 255; see also Freud, "Formulations on the Two Principles of Mental Functioning" (1911), in *SE* 12: 222.
82. Freud, *Three Essays*, p. 148; see also his *Drei Abhandlungen zur Sexualtheorie*, in *GW* 5: 46. Freud also used this expression to describe the relationship between idea and affect: see *The Interpretation of Dreams*, p. 462, and *Die Traumdeutung*, in *GW* 2/3: 464.
83. Freud, *The Interpretation of Dreams*, pp. 266–267.
84. Ibid., p. 256; see also Freud, *Introductory Lectures on Psycho-Analysis*, pp. 187–190.
85. See Freud, "Some Psychical Consequences of the Anatomical Distinction between the Sexes" (1925), in *SE* 19: 251, and Freud, "Female Sexuality," pp. 225–226.
86. Freud, *The Interpretation of Dreams*, pp. 256, 257, 258, 261, 264 (emphasis in the original).
87. Ibid., p. 264. For an earlier and very similar discussion of *Oedipus Rex*, see Freud to Fliess, October 15, 1897, *F/F Letters*, p. 272.
88. Freud, *The Interpretation of Dreams*, p. 261; see also Freud, "Draft N" (enclosed with letter of May 31, 1897), in *F/F Letters*, p. 250.
89. Freud, "Analysis of a Phobia in a Five-Year-Old-Boy" (1909), in *SE* 10: 42, 111; see also Freud to Jung, December 11, 1908, *F/J Letters*, p. 186.
90. Freud, *Three Essays*, p. 189.
91. Freud, "Analysis of a Phobia," pp. 118–119.
92. Freud, *Three Essays*, pp. 157, 158 (emphasis in the original).
93. Freud, "On the Sexual Theories of Children" (1908) in *SE* 9: 220–221 (emphasis in the original).

94. Freud, "Analysis of a Phobia," p. 112 (emphasis in the original).

95. Ibid., pp. 79–81 (emphasis in the original).

96. Freud, "Draft H. Paranoia" (enclosed with letter of January 24, 1895), in *F/F Letters,* p. 109.

97. Freud, *Inhibitions, Symptoms and Anxiety* (1926), in *SE* 20: 106.

98. Freud to Jung, December 11, 1908, *The Freud/Jung Letters,* p. 186; see also Freud, "'A Child Is Being Beaten': A Contribution to the Study of the Origin of Sexual Perversions" (1919), in *SE* 17: 204.

99. Freud, "Notes upon a Case of Obsessional Neurosis" (1909), in *SE* 10: 187.

100. The eminent Julius Wagner von Jauregg was one of the many physicians consulted: see Freud, *L'Homme aux rats: Journal d'une analyse,* trans. Elza Ribeiro Hawalka (Paris: Presses Universitaires de France, 1974), pp. 46–47.

101. "Why don't you say it (aloud)?" turned up in Daniel Paul Schreber, *Memoirs of My Nervous Illness,* trans. Ida Macalpine and Richard A. Hunter (Cambridge, Mass.: Harvard University Press, 1988), pp. 70*n*, 121, and Jung commented on the appropriateness of this question for psychoanalysis: see Jung to Freud, September 29, 1910, *F/J Letters,* p. 356.

102. Freud, "Notes upon a Case of Obsessional Neurosis," pp. 166–167 (emphasis in the original).

103. Ibid., p. 167.

104. Freud, *L'Homme aux rats,* p. 46.

105. See October 30 and November 6, 1907, *Minutes of the Vienna Psychoanalytic Society* 1: 227–241; November 20, 1907, ibid. 1: 246; January 22, 1908, ibid., 1: 287; April 8, 1908, ibid., 1: 370–371.

106. Freud to Jung, April 19, 1908, *F/J Letters,* p. 141.

107. Freud to Jung, April 19, 1908, ibid., p. 141.

108. Ernest Jones, *The Life and Work of Sigmund Freud,* vol. 2, *Years of Maturity 1901–1919* (New York: Basic Books, 1955), p. 42.

109. Freud to Jung, June 3, 1909, *F/J Letters,* p. 227, and June 30, 1909, p. 238.

110. Freud, "Notes upon a Case of Obsessional Neurosis," pp. 155, 159*n*. Elza Ribeiro Hawalka has transcribed, in meticulous fashion, the complete German text of Freud's process notes (the text in the *SE* 10: 253–318 is incomplete) and has added a facing French translation, notes, and commentaries: see Freud, *L'Homme aux rats.*

111. Steven Marcus, *Freud and the Culture of Psychoanalysis: Studies in the Transition from Victorian Humanism to Modernity* (New York: Norton, 1984), p. 164.

112. Freud to Jung, June 3, 1909, *F/J Letters,* p. 227.

113. Freud, "Notes upon a Case of Obsessional Neurosis," p. 155.

114. The German is "Vereinfachung": see Freud, "Bemerkungen über einen Fall von Zwangsneurose," in *GW* 7: 454; see also his *Das Ich und das Es*, in *GW* 13: 261.
115. Ibid., pp. 237, 238, 239.
116. Ibid., p. 239*n*.
117. For biographical information on Lanzer, as well as a thorough examination of the discrepancies between the process notes and the published text, see Patrick J. Mahony, *Freud and the Rat Man* (New Haven: Yale University Press, 1986).
118. Freud, "Notes upon a Case of Obsessional Neurosis," pp. 174–175, 200–201, 294 (emphasis in the original).
119. Freud to Jung, October 17, 1909, *F/J Letters*, p. 255. Freud may have exaggerated the length of the treatment: see Mahony, *Freud and the Rat Man*, pp. 69–70.
120. Freud, "Notes upon a Case of Obsessional Neurosis," pp. 158, 160–162, 178–180 (emphasis in the original).
121. Ibid., p. 182 (emphasis in the original).
122. October 30, and November 6, 1907, *Minutes of the Vienna Psychoanalytic Society* 1: 236.
123. Freud, "Notes upon a Case of Obsessional Neurosis," pp. 203–205, 261; see also Freud, *L'Homme aux rats*, pp. 97–103.
124. Freud, "Fragment of an Analysis," p. 12.
125. Freud, "Notes upon a Case of Obsessional Neurosis," pp. 205–206.
126. Ibid., p. 207*n*.
127. Ibid., p. 307.
128. Freud, "A Special Type of Choice of Object Made by Men (Contributions to the Psychology of Love I)" (1910), in *SE* 11: 166, 168–169, 170, 171.
129. Freud, "Notes upon a Case of Obsessional Neurosis," p. 301; see also his "Sexual Theories of Children," p. 226, and "A Special Type of Choice of Object," p. 170.
130. Freud, "Notes upon a Case of Obsessional Neurosis," p. 208*n;* see also his *Introductory Lectures on Psycho-Analysis*, p. 337, and "An Autobiographical Study," p. 55.
131. Freud, "Notes upon a Case of Obsessional Neurosis," p. 208*n*.
132. See Freud, *Introductory Lectures on Psycho-Analysis*, p. 368.
133. Freud, "Psycho-Analytic Notes on an Autobiographical Account of a Case of Paranoia (Dementia Paranoides)" (1911), in *SE* 12: 68–69.
134. Ibid., pp. 70, 71 (emphasis in the original).
135. Ibid., p. 72.
136. Freud had earlier linked paranoia with a return to an auto-erotic state: see Freud to Fliess, December 9, 1899, *F/F Letters*, p. 390. Karl Abraham had postulated a similar regression in cases of dementia praecox: see Karl Abraham, "The Psycho-Sexual Differences between Hysteria and Demen-

tia Praecox" (1908), in *Selected Papers of Karl Abraham,* trans. Douglas Bryan and Alix Strachey (London: Hogarth Press, 1927; reprint, London: Karnac, Maresfield Reprints, 1979), pp. 64–79. Freud acknowledged a debt to Abraham: see Freud to Abraham, December 18, 1910, *F/A Letters,* p. 97.

137. Freud, *Three Essays,* pp. 222, 225.

138. Freud, "Psycho-Analytic Notes on . . . a Case of Paranoia," p. 72.

139. Freud, "Mourning and Melancholia" (1917), in *SE* 14: 249; see also his *Group Psychology and the Analysis of the Ego* (1921), in *SE* 18: 109.

140. November 10, 1909, *Minutes of the Vienna Psychoanalytic Society* 2: 312.

141. Freud to Jung, October 17, 1909, *F/J Letters,* p. 255.

142. Freud, *Leonardo da Vinci and a Memory of His Childhood* (1910), in *SE* 11: 134, 135.

143. Freud to Fliess, October 9, 1898, *F/F Letters,* p. 331.

144. Freud, "Contribution to a Questionnaire on Reading" (1907), in *SE* 9: 246.

145. Freud, *Leonardo,* pp. 71, 72–73, 105.

146. Freud to Jung, October 17, 1909, *F/J Letters,* p. 255.

147. Leonardo da Vinci, *Codex Atlanticus* (Milan: Giovanni Piumati, 1894–1904), F.65 v., quoted in Freud, *Leonardo,* p. 82.

148. Freud, *Leonardo,* p. 84.

149. Ibid., pp. 86, 91, 94, 107 (emphasis in the original).

150. Ibid., pp. 107, 108, 114, 116–117; see also Freud, *Group Psychology and the Analysis of the Ego,* pp. 108–109.

151. Freud, *Leonardo,* pp. 98, 100, 102 (emphasis in the original).

152. December 1, 1909, *Minutes of the Vienna Psychoanalytic Society* 3: 343.

153. See Freud, "On Narcissism: An Introduction" (1914), in *SE* 14: 88; see also May 26, 1909, *Minutes of the Vienna Psychoanalytic Society* 3: 258, and Freud, *Three Essays,* p. 144*n*.

154. Freud, *Leonardo,* p. 100.

155. Freud, "From the History of an Infantile Neurosis" (1918), in *SE* 17: 7; see also p. 8.

156. Ibid., p. 17.

157. "The Memoirs of the Wolf-Man," trans. Muriel Gardiner, in Gardiner, ed., *The Wolf-Man by the Wolf-Man,* p. 7. I have relied on these memoirs for biographical information as well as on Patrick J. Mahony, *Cries of the Wolf Man* (New York: International Universities Press, 1984).

158. Freud, "History of an Infantile Neurosis," p. 7. For a discussion of conflicting statements about Sergei's age at the time of the infection, see Mahony, *The Wolf Man,* p. 20*n*.

159. "The Memoirs of the Wolf-Man," pp. 83, 138.

160. Freud, "History of an Infantile Neurosis," p. 118.

161. Freud, "Remembering, Repeating and Working-Through," p. 153.

162. Karin Obholzer, *The Wolf-Man Sixty Years Later: Conversations with Freud's Controversial Patient,* trans. Michael Shaw (London: Routledge and Kegan Paul, 1982), p. 104.

163. Ibid., p. 231; see also Freud, "Analysis Terminable and Interminable" (1937), in *SE* 23: 217–218.

164. "The Memoirs of the Wolf-Man," p. 111.

165. Freud, "History of an Infantile Neurosis," pp. 8–9.

166. Ibid., p. 99; see also November 17, 1909, *Minutes of the Vienna Psychoanalytic Society* 2: 322, and February 25, 1914, 4: 231; Freud, *Introductory Lectures on Psycho-Analysis,* pp. 363–364.

167. Freud, "History of an Infantile Neurosis," pp. 29, 33 (emphasis in the original); see also "Letters Pertaining to Freud's 'History of an Infantile Neurosis,'" *The Psychoanalytic Quarterly* 26 (1957): 449–460.

168. Freud, "History of an Infantile Neurosis," pp. 33, 42*n.*

169. Ibid., p. 97.

170. Ibid., pp. 33, 34, 35 (emphasis in the original).

171. Ibid., pp. 36–37 (emphasis in the original).

172. Ibid., pp. 30–31, 42 (emphasis in the original).

173. Ibid., pp. 36, 70, 112.

174. Ibid., pp. 24, 26, 27, 28; see also Freud, "'A Child Is Being Beaten,'" p. 198.

175. Freud, "History of an Infantile Neurosis," pp. 24, 25, 45*n*, 46, 47.

176. Freud, *Inhibition, Symptoms and Anxiety,* p. 108.

177. Freud, "History of an Infantile Neurosis," pp. 16, 32.

178. Obholzer, *The Wolf-Man Sixty Years Later,* p. 4.

179. Freud, "Mourning and Melancholia" (1917), in *SE* 14: 248–249 (emphasis in the original); see Freud, *The Ego and the Id,* p. 30.

180. See Freud, "On Narcissism," p. 74.

181. See Freud, "History of an Infantile Neurosis," pp. 117–118.

4. Modes of Conversation

1. Michel Foucault, *The History of Sexuality,* vol. 1, *An Introduction,* trans. Robert Hurley (New York: Vintage/Random House, 1980), pp. 59, 61–62.

2. See John Forrester, *The Seductions of Psychoanalysis: Freud, Lacan and Derrida* (Cambridge: Cambridge University Press, 1990), pp. 287–316; see also Hubert L. Dreyfus and Paul Rabinow, *Michel Foucault: Beyond Structuralism and Hermeneutics,* 2d ed. (Chicago: University of Chicago Press, 1983), pp. 168–183. For Freud's comments on the comparison between psychoanalysis and confession, see Josef Breuer and Sigmund Freud, *Studies on Hysteria* (1893–1895), in *SE* 2: 282; Freud, *The Question*

of Lay Analysis: Conversations with an Impartial Person (1926), in *SE* 20: 189; Freud, *An Outline of Psycho-Analysis* (1940), in *SE* 23: 174.

3. Freud to Stefan Zweig, June 2, 1932, *Letters of Sigmund Freud,* ed. Ernst L. Freud, trans. Tania and James Stern (New York: Basic Books, 1960), p. 413.

4. See Breuer and Freud, *Studies on Hysteria,* p. 40*n;* see Freud: "On the History of the Psycho-Analytic Movement" (1914), in *SE* 14: 12; "Josef Breuer" (1925), in *SE* 19: 280; "An Autobiographical Study" (1925), in *SE* 20: 20–21; and *The Question of Lay Analysis,* p. 225.

5. Ernest Jones, *The Life and Work of Sigmund Freud,* vol. 1, *The Formative Years and the Great Discoveries 1856–1900* (New York: Basic Books, 1953), pp. 224–225.

6. Freud, *Introductory Lectures on Psycho-Analysis* (1916–1917), in *SE* 16: 441–442 (emphasis in the original).

7. Ibid., p. 442.

8. Freud, *An Outline of Psycho-Analysis,* p. 176.

9. Freud, "The Dynamics of Transference" (1912), in *SE* 12: 107.

10. Freud, *An Outline of Psycho-Analysis,* p. 176.

11. Freud, *The Question of Lay Analysis,* p. 225.

12. Freud, "Observations on Transference-Love (Further Recommendations on the Technique of Psycho-Analysis III)" (1915), in *SE* 12: 162.

13. Freud, *The Question of Lay Analysis,* p. 226.

14. Freud, "Transference-Love," p. 160.

15. Ibid., pp. 169–170.

16. See Freud to Martha Bernays, November 4, 1883, quoted in Forrester, *The Seductions of Psychoanalysis,* pp. 19–20.

17. Breuer and Freud, *Studies on Hysteria,* pp. 106, 260.

18. Ibid., pp. 108, 109–110; see also Freud, "An Autobiographical Study," pp. 27–28.

19. Breuer and Freud, *Studies on Hysteria,* pp. 110, 270.

20. For slightly differing accounts of Freud's technique, see ibid., pp. 110–111, 270–272.

21. Ibid., pp. 113–114.

22. Ibid., pp. 114, 115.

23. Ibid., pp. 116, 117 (emphasis in the original).

24. Ibid., pp. 118, 119.

25. Ibid., p. 120.

26. Ibid.

27. Ibid.

28. Ibid., p. 121.

29. Freud, "Fragment of an Analysis of a Case of Hysteria" (1905), in *SE* 7: 23–24 (emphasis in the original).

30. Breuer and Freud, *Studies on Hysteria,* p. 260.

31. Freud, "My Views on the Part Played by Sexuality in the Aetiology of the Neuroses" (1906), in *SE* 7: 274, 278. Freud first used the term "psycho-analysis" in 1896: see his "Heredity and the Aetiology of the Neuroses" (1896), in *SE* 3: 151, and "Further Remarks on the Neuro-Psychoses of Defence" (1896), in *SE* 3: 162.

32. Freud, "Fragment of an Analysis," p. 12. See also Freud, "An Autobiographical Study," pp. 40–41.

33. Freud, "Freud's Psycho-Analytic Procedure" (1904), in *SE* 7: 250; see also his *The Interpretation of Dreams* (1900), in *SE* 4: 101.

34. Freud, "Notes upon a Case of Obsessional Neurosis" (1909), in *SE* 10: 159 (emphasis in the original); see also his "On Beginning the Treatment (Further Recommendations on the Technique of Psycho-Analysis I)" (1913), in *SE* 12: 134–135, and *The Question of Lay Analysis,* p. 218.

35. Breuer and Freud, *Studies on Hysteria,* p. 63.

36. Ibid., p. 271.

37. Freud, "Fragment of an Analysis," pp. 18, 35.

38. Freud, *The Interpretation of Dreams,* p. 100.

39. Freud, "Fragment of an Analysis," p. 10.

40. Ibid., p. 69n.

41. Ibid., pp. 20, 68–70.

42. Ibid., p. 70.

43. Ibid., pp. 75, 76.

44. Ibid., pp. 82; here Freud broached the third, the fragmentary interpretation of Dora's cough mentioned in chapter 3, note 105.

45. Ibid., p. 87; see also ibid., p. 76n.

46. Ibid., p. 94 (emphasis in the original).

47. Ibid., pp. 97, 98 (emphasis in the original).

48. Ibid., pp. 98, 99–100 (emphasis in the original).

49. Ibid., pp. 100, 103–104.

50. Ibid., pp. 105, 106–108, 109 (emphasis in the original).

51. Ibid., p. 109.

52. Breuer and Freud, *Studies on Hysteria,* pp. 302–303; see also Freud, *The Interpretation of Dreams,* pp. 531–532.

53. Freud, "Fragment of an Analysis," p. 116.

54. Ibid., pp. 73–74.

55. Ibid., p. 119.

56. Ibid., p. 118.

57. Ibid., p. 119.

58. There is a considerable feminist literature directed at uncovering transferences that Freud did not appreciate—transferences which cast him in a female role. Among the most suggestive commentaries are: Toril Moi, "Representation of Patriarchy: Sexuality and Epistemology in Freud's Dora," in Charles Bernheimer and Claire Kahane, eds., *In Dora's Case:*

Freud—Hysteria—Feminism (New York: Columbia University Press, 1985), pp. 181–199; Neil Hertz, "Dora's Secrets, Freud's Techniques," in ibid., pp. 221–242; Jane Collins, J. Ray Green, Mary Lydon, Mark Sachner, and Eleanor Honig Skoller, "Questioning the Unconscious: The Dora Archive," in ibid., pp. 243–253; Forrester, *The Seductions of Psychoanalysis*, pp. 49–61. For useful discussions of transference more generally in this case, see Hyman Muslin and Merton Gill, "Transference in the Dora Case," *JAPA* 26 (1978): 311–328, and Phillip McCaffrey, *Freud and Dora: The Artful Dream* (New Brunswick, N.J.: Rutgers University Press, 1984).

59. Freud, "Fragment of an Analysis," pp. 58, 120.

60. Ibid., p. 120*n*.

61. Freud, "The Psychogenesis of a Case of Homosexuality in a Woman" (1920), in *SE* 18: 147–148, 150, 151, 152.

62. Ibid., pp. 152, 155, 156. "The specially intense bond with her latest love had still another basis which the girl discovered quite easily one day. Her lady's slender figure, severe beauty, and downright manner reminded her of . . . [a] brother who was a little older than herself. Her latest choice corresponded, therefore, not only to her feminine ideal but also to her masculine ideal." (ibid., p. 156).

63. Ibid., p. 153.

64. Ibid., pp. 156, 157 (emphasis in the original). Compare Freud to Ferenczi, March 3, 1912.

65. Freud, "Psychogenesis of a Case of Homosexuality," p. 164.

66. Freud to Fliess, August 14, 1897, *F/F Letters,* p. 261.

67. Freud, *The Interpretation of Dreams,* p. xxvi. On Freud's self-analysis, see Didier Anzieu, *Freud's Self-Analysis,* trans. Peter Graham (London: Hogarth Press, 1986); see also Edith Buxbaum, "Freud's Dream Interpretation in the Light of His Letters to Fliess," *Bulletin of the Menninger Clinic* 15 (1951): 197–212; Suzanne Cassirer Bernfeld, "Discussion of Buxbaum, 'Freud's Dream Interpretation in the Light of His Letters to Fliess,'" *Bulletin of the Menninger Clinic* 16 (1952): 70–72; Jones, *Sigmund Freud* 1: 319–327; Max Schur, *Freud: Living and Dying* (New York: International Universities Press, 1972), pp. 63–222; Patrick Mahony, "Friendship and Its Discontents," *Contemporary Psychoanalysis* 15 (1979): 55–109.

68. Freud, *The Interpretation of Dreams,* pp. 106*n*, 107 (emphasis and ellipses in the original). For variants on the Strachey translation, see Erik Homburger Erikson, "The Dream Specimen of Psychoanalysis," *JAPA* 2 (1954): 24–27, and Patrick J. Mahony, "Towards a Formalist Approach to Dreams," *IRP* 4 (1977): 85–86. The commentaries on the dream I have found most useful, in addition to the above two, are: Harry C. Leavitt, "A Biological and Teleological Study of 'Irma's Injection' Dream," *Psychoanalytic Review* 43 (1956): 440–447; Max Schur, "Some Additional 'Day

Residues' of the 'Specimen Dream of Psychoanalysis,'" in R. M. Loewen-stein, L. M. Newman, M. Schur, and A. J. Solnit, eds., *Psychoanalysis—A General Psychology: Essays in Honor of Heinz Hartmann* (New York: Inter-national Universities Press, 1966), pp. 45–85; Alexander Grinstein, *On Sigmund Freud's Dreams* (Detroit, Mich.: Wayne State University Press, 1968), pp. 21–46; R. Greenberg and C. Pearlman, "If Only Freud Knew: A Reconsideration of Psychoanalytic Dream Theory," *IRP* 5 (1978): 71–75; Adam Kuper and Alan A. Stone, "The Dream of Irma's Injection: A Structural Analysis," *The American Journal of Psychiatry* 139 (1982): 1225–1234; Frank R. Hartman, "A Reappraisal of the Emma Episode and the Specimen Dream," *JAPA* 31 (1983): 555–585; Anzieu, *Freud's Self-Analysis,* pp. 131–155.

69. Freud, *The Interpretation of Dreams,* pp. 106, 108.
70. Ibid., pp. 106, 108.
71. Ibid., pp. 114, 115, 119 (emphasis in the original).
72. Ibid., p. 595.
73. Ibid., p. 116; see also Sigmund Freud, "Project for a Scientific Psychol-ogy" (1950), in *SE* 1: 341–342.
74. Freud to Abraham, January 9, 1908, *F/A Letters,* p. 20.
75. Freud, *The Interpretation of Dreams,* pp. 116–117.
76. Ibid., p. 117.
77. "Irma" was not Emma Eckstein; her real name was Anna Hammerschlag Lichtheim: see Jeffrey Moussaieff Masson, *The Assault on Truth: Freud's Suppression of the Seduction Theory* (New York: Farrar, Straus and Giroux, 1984), p. 205*n*1.
78. Freud to Fliess, May 15, 1895, *F/F Letters,* p. 130.
79. See Freud, "Draft I. Migraine: Established Points," (undated, ?October 8, 1895), in ibid., pp. 142–144, and Freud to Fliess, May 4, 1896, ibid., p. 186.
80. Freud to Fliess, January 24, 1895, ibid., p. 107.
81. Freud to Fliess, March 4, 1895, ibid., pp. 113–114.
82. Freud to Fliess, March 8, 1895, ibid., pp. 116–117.
83. Freud to Fliess, March 8, 1895, ibid., p. 117, and April 20, 1895, p. 125. Not until May 25, 1895, did Freud report that Emma was "finally doing very well" and that he had "succeeded in once more alleviating her weak-ness in walking," which had "set in again": Freud to Fliess, May 25, 1895, ibid., p. 130.
84. Freud to Fliess, February 13, 1896, ibid., p. 172. For a tendentious ac-count of Freud's continued loyalty to Fliess and its repercussions on psy-choanalytic theory, see Masson, *The Assault on Truth,* pp. 55–106.
85. See Freud to Fliess, June 12, 1900, *F/F Letters,* p. 417, and June 18, 1900, p. 419.
86. I am assuming that when Freud asked Fliess to return "the dream exam-

ples" he had sent to him, the Irma dream was among them: Freud to Fliess, December 12, 1897, ibid., p. 286; compare the variant translation in Freud, *The Origins of Psychoanalysis, Letters to Wilhelm Fliess, Drafts and Notes: 1887–1902,* ed. Marie Bonaparte, Anna Freud, and Ernst Kris, trans. Eric Mosbacher and James Strachey (New York: Basic Books, 1954), p. 238. The German is : "Darf ich Dich bitten, mir die eingeschickten Traumbeispiele (insoweit sie auf separaten Blättern standen) nach Breslau mitzubringen?" *Sigmund Freud: Briefe an Wilhelm Fliess 1887–1904,* ed. Jeffrey Moussaieff Masson, assisted by Michael Schröter and Gerhard Fichtner (Frankfurt: S. Fischer, 1986), p. 311.

87. Freud to Fliess, November 14, 1897, *F/F Letters,* p. 281.

88. Freud to Fliess, April 20, 1895, p. 125, and July 24, 1895, p. 134. Freud had put himself in Fliess's hands for both treatment of his cardiac symptoms and cauterizations of his nose; for Fliess as Freud's physician, see Schur, *Freud: Living and Dying,* pp. 40–138.

89. For Freud's acknowledgment of the homoerotic element in his relationship to Fliess, see Freud to Fliess, May 7, 1900, *F/F Letters,* p. 412, and August 7, 1908, p. 447; see also Freud to Ferenczi, October 6, 1910, quoted in Ernest Jones, *The Life and Work of Sigmund Freud,* vol. 2, *Years of Maturity 1901–1919* (New York: Basic Books, 1955), p. 83.

90. Frank J. Sulloway, *Freud, Biologist of the Mind: Beyond the Psychoanalytic Legend* (New York: Basic Books, 1979), pp. 139, 140.

91. The two men had obviously discussed bisexuality before their Breslau meeting: see Freud to Fliess, December 6, 1896, *F/F Letters,* p. 212. Periodicity theory also led Fliess to bilaterality, the view that "left and right were as different and as complementary as the two sexes": Anzieu, *Freud's Self-Analysis,* p. 256; see also Freud to Fliess, December 29, 1897, *F/F Letters,* p. 290, and January 4, 1898, p. 292. Alone among Fliess's theories, bilaterality provoked an immediate skeptical response in Freud.

92. Freud to Fliess, October 15, 1897, *F/F Letters,* p. 272, and December 22, 1897, p. 287.

93. Freud to Fliess, September 21, 1897, ibid., p. 266; February 9, 1898, p. 298; and March 24, 1898, p. 305.

94. Freud, *The Interpretation of Dreams,* p. 172 (emphasis in the original).

95. Freud to Fliess, March 10, 1898, *F/F Letters,* pp. 301–302.

96. The most useful commentaries on the dream are Grinstein, *On Sigmund Freud's Dreams,* pp. 47–68, and Anzieu, *Freud's Self-Analysis,* pp. 278–294.

97. Freud, *The Interpretation of Dreams,* pp. 170, 171. For Freud's subsequent (1914) comments on eye-symbolism, the blinding of Oedipus, and castration, see ibid., p. 398*n*.

98. Ibid., pp. 165, 169, 282 (emphasis in the original).

99. Ibid., p. 169 (emphasis in the original).

100. Ibid., p. 172 (emphasis in the original).

101. Ibid., pp. 171, 172, 173 (emphasis in the original).

102. Ibid., pp. 173, 467.

103. Ibid., p. 467.

104. Freud to Fliess, January 16, 1898, *F/F Letters,* p. 294, and January 22, 1898, p. 296.

105. I have inferred the date from Anzieu, *Freud's Self-Analysis,* pp. 270–272.

106. Ry. [Benjamin Rischawy?], review of *Die Beziehungen zwischen Nase und weiblichen Geschlechtsorganen,* by Wilhelm Fliess, *Wiener klinische Rundschau, Organ für die gesamte praktische Heilkunde sowie für die Interessen des ärtzlichen Standes* (April 10, 1898), quoted and translated in Grinstein, *On Sigmund Freud's Dreams,* p. 249.

107. See the dream of "Goethe's Attack on Herr M.": Freud, *The Interpretation of Dreams,* pp. 439–441, 448–449.

108. Freud to Fliess, May 18, 1898, *F/F Letters,* p. 313.

109. Freud to Fliess, October 23, 1898, ibid., p. 332.

110. Freud, *The Interpretation of Dreams,* p. 421 (emphasis in the original). For useful commentaries on the dream see Grinstein, *On Sigmund Freud's Dreams,* pp. 282–316; Schur, *Freud: Living and Dying,* pp. 153–171; Max Schur, "The Background to Freud's 'Disturbance' on the Acropolis," in Mark Kanzer and Jules Glenn, eds., *Freud and His Self-Analysis* (New York: Jason Aronson, 1979), pp. 117–134; Anzieu, *Freud's Self-Analysis,* pp. 375–388.

111. Freud, *The Interpretation of Dreams,* p. 423.

112. Ibid., pp. 521–522, 523.

113. Ibid., pp. 480–481, 481*n.*

114. Freud to Fliess, November 2, 1896, *F/F Letters,* p. 202. For a slightly different version, see Freud, *The Interpretation of Dreams,* pp. 317–318.

115. See Breuer and Freud, *Studies on Hysteria,* pp. 163, 164*n.*

116. See Freud, *The Interpretation of Dreams,* p. 423*n.*

117. See Schur, *Freud: Living and Dying,* p. 119, and Peter Gay, *Freud: A Life for Our Time* (New York: Norton, 1988) p. 8. Jones gives a different chronology: see Jones, *Freud* 1: 7.

118. Freud to Fliess, October 3, 1897, *F/F Letters,* p. 268.

119. Freud, *The Interpretation of Dreams,* p. 230; see also Freud to Fliess, November 6, 1898, *F/F Letters,* p. 334.

120. Freud to Fliess, May 28, 1899, *F/F Letters,* p. 353, and August 1, 1899, p. 363.

121. Freud, *The Interpretation of Dreams,* p. 425.

122. Ibid., pp. 483–484 (emphasis in the original). For a less full version of the fight with John, see pp. 424–425; see also p. 513.

123. Ibid., p. 424.

124. William Shakespeare, *Julius Caesar* (iii, 2), quoted in Freud, *The Interpre-*

tation of Dreams, p. 424. Freud associated to the same lines in writing about Ernst Lanzer: see Freud, "Notes upon a Case of Obsessional Neurosis," p. 180.

125. Freud to Fliess, October 3, 1897, *F/F Letters,* p. 268.

126. Freud, *The Interpretation of Dreams,* pp. 483, 485.

127. Freud to Fliess, September 21, 1899, *F/F Letters,* p. 374.

128. See Freud to Fliess, September 6, 1899, ibid., p. 370; see also Freud to Jung, February 17, 1911, *F/J Letters,* p. 395.

129. Freud, *The Interpretation of Dreams,* p. 484 (emphasis in the original).

130. Freud, *The Psychopathology of Everyday Life* (1901), in *SE* 6: 143–144.

131. Freud to Fliess, March 15, 1898, *F/F Letters,* p. 303.

132. Freud, *The Interpretation of Dreams,* p. 331. For a discussion of the date this dream was dreamt and interpreted, see Anzieu, *Freud's Self-Analysis,* pp. 322–324.

133. Freud, *The Interpretation of Dreams,* p. 606.

134. Freud to Fliess, August 1, 1899, *F/F Letters,* p. 364.

135. Freud to Fliess, January 30, 1901, ibid., p. 434; August 7, 1901, p. 448; and September 19, 1901, p. 450.

136. Fliess to Freud, July 20, 1904, ibid., p. 463. Among the many accounts of the Weininger-Swoboda episode, the fullest is Vincent Brome, *Freud and His Early Circle: The Struggle of Psycho-Analysis* (London: Heinemann, 1967), pp. 1–13.

137. Freud to Fliess, July 27, 1904, *F/F Letters,* p. 466.

138. Freud, "Constructions in Analysis," (1937), in *SE* 23: 257, 261, 262, 263, 265 (emphasis in the original).

139. Freud, "Notes upon a Case of Obsessional Neurosis," pp. 202, 263.

140. Ibid., pp. 264–265.

141. Ibid., pp. 207–208.

142. Freud, "On Beginning the Treatment," p. 140.

143. Freud, "Fragment of an Analysis," p. 109.

144. Freud, *Introductory Lectures on Psycho-Analysis,* p. 437.

145. Freud, "On Beginning the Treatment," pp. 139, 140.

146. Freud, "Notes upon a Case of Obsessional Neurosis," p. 175; see also his "Analysis of a Phobia in a Five-Year-Old Boy" (1909), in *SE* 10: 104.

147. Freud, "Notes upon a Case of Obsessional Neurosis," pp. 175–176.

148. Freud, *Introductory Lectures on Psycho-Analysis,* p. 437.

149. November 6, 1907, *Minutes of the Vienna Psychoanalytic Society,* ed. Herman Nunberg and Ernst Federn, trans. M. Nunberg, 4 vols. (New York: International Universities Press, 1962–1975) 1: 227.

150. Ibid.

151. Freud, "Notes upon a Case of Obsessional Neurosis," pp. 177, 178 (emphasis in the original).

152. Ibid., pp. 159, 172 (emphasis in the original).

153. Ibid., pp. 159–160, 160*n*.
154. Freud, "The Dynamics of Transference," p. 105.
155. See Martin H. Stein, "The Unobjectionable Part of the Transference," *JAPA* 29 (1981): 869–892. The commentaries on Freud's handling of the transference in Ernst's case that I have found most useful are: Ernst Kris, "Ego Psychologgy and Interpretation in Psychoanalytic Therapy," *The Psychoanalytic Quarterly* 20 (1951): 15–30; Elizabeth Zetzel, "1965: Additional Notes upon a Case of Obsessional Neurosis: Freud 1909," *IJP* 47 (1966): 123–129; Béla Grunberger, "Some Reflections on the Rat Man," *IJP* 47 (1966): 160–167; René Major, "The Language of Interpretation," *IRP* 1 (1974): 425–435; Jerome S. Beigler, "A Commentary on Freud's Treatment of the Rat Man," *Annual of Psychoanalysis* 3 (1975): 271–285; Samuel D. Lipton, "The Advantages of Freud's Technique as Shown in His Analysis of the Rat Man," *IJP* 58 (1977): 255–273; Samuel D. Lipton, "An Addendum to 'The Advantages of Freud's Technique as Shown in His Analysis of the Rat Man,'" *IJP* 60 (1979): 215–216; Hyman L. Muslin, "Transference in the Rat Man Case: The Transference in Transition," *JAPA* 27 (1979): 561–578; Mark Kanzer, "The Transference Neurosis of the Rat Man," in Mark Kanzer and Jules Glenn, eds., *Freud and His Patients* (New York: Jason Aronson, 1980), pp. 137–143; Stanley J. Weiss, "Reflections and Speculations on the Psychoanalysis of the Rat Man," in ibid., pp. 203–214; Robert J. Langs, "The Misalliance Dimension in the Case of the Rat Man," in ibid., pp. 215–231; Mark Kanzer, "Freud's 'Human Influence' on the Rat Man," in ibid., pp. 232–240; K. H. Blacker and Ruth Abraham, "The Rat Man Revisited: Comments on Maternal Influences," *The International Journal of Psychoanalytic Psychotherapy* 9 (1982): 705–727.
156. Freud, *The Interpretation of Dreams*, pp. 562, 563.
157. Freud, "Fragment of an Analysis," p. 116; see also Merton M. Gill, "The Analysis of the Transference," *JAPA* 27 (suppl.) (1979): 263–288.
158. Freud, "Analysis Terminable and Interminable" (1937), in *SE* 23: 221–222. See also Ferenczi to Freud, January 17, 1930; Freud to Ferenczi, January 20, 1930; Ferenczi to Freud, February 14, 1930.
159. Freud, "Notes upon a Case of Obsessional Neurosis," pp. 289, 292.
160. Ibid., pp. 166, 169 (emphasis in the original).
161. Ibid. p. 284.
162. Ibid., pp. 199, 200 (emphasis in the original).
163. Freud to Jung, October 17, 1909, *F/J Letters*, p. 255.
164. Freud, "Notes upon a Case of Obsessional Neurosis," p. 167 (emphasis in the original).
165. Freud, "On Beginning the Treatment," p. 140; see also his "'Wild' Psycho-Analysis" (1910), in *SE* 11: 226, and *The Question of Lay Analysis*, p. 220.
166. Freud, "Notes upon a Case of Obsessional Neurosis," p. 167.

167. Ibid., p. 167 (emphasis in the original).

168. Ibid., pp. 213, 214.

169. Ibid., pp. 209, 213, 307.

170. Ibid., pp. 170–171, 173.

171. Ibid., pp. 215–216.

172. Ibid., pp. 282, 283.

173. Ibid., p. 207*n.*

174. See Allan D. Rosenblatt, "Epilogue: Transference Neurosis: Phenomenon in Search of a Referent," *Psychoanalytic Inquiry* 7 (1987): 577–603.

175. Freud, "Notes upon a Case of Obsessional Neurosis," p. 292; see also Freud, *L'Homme aux Rats: Journal d'une analyse,* trans. Elza Ribero Hawalka (Paris, Presses Universitaires de France, 1974), p. 179*n.*

176. Freud, "Remembering, Repeating and Working-Through (Further Recommendations on the Technique of Psycho-Analysis II)" (1914), in *SE* 12: 154.

177. Freud, *Introductory Lectures on Psycho-Analysis,* p. 444; see also pp. 454–455.

178. Freud, *The Interpretation of Dreams,* p. 184 (emphasis in the original).

179. Freud, *Beyond the Pleasure Principle* (1920), in *SE* 18: 18 (emphasis in the original).

180. Freud, "Fragment of an Analysis," p. 117.

181. Freud, "Notes upon a Case of Obsessional Neurosis," p. 176.

182. Freud, "The Dynamics of Transference," p. 108 (emphasis in the original); see also Freud, "Notes upon a Case of Obsessional Neurosis," p. 182.

183. Freud, "Remembering, Repeating and Working-Through," p. 152.

184. See Freud, "Notes upon a Case of Obsessional Neurosis," pp. 164, 248–249, 278.

185. Freud, *Introductory Lectures on Psycho-Analysis,* p. 446.

186. Ibid., pp. 450, 451 (emphasis in the original); see also Freud, *The Question of Lay Analysis,* pp. 190, 225.

187. Freud, *Introductory Lectures on Psycho-Analysis,* p. 449 (emphasis in the original).

188. Ibid., pp. 446–447.

189. Freud to Fliess, August 7, 1901, *F/F Letters,* p. 447.

190. See Freud, "The Future Prospects of Psycho-Analytic Therapy" (1910), in *SE* 11: 144, and Freud, "Transference-Love," pp. 160, 165, 169. See also Robert L. Tyson, "Countertransference Evolution in Theory and Practice," *JAPA* 34 (1986): 251–274.

191. Freud to Abraham, December 26, 1908, *F/A Letters,* p. 63; see also Freud to Jung, June 7, 1909, *F/J Letters,* p. 231. Compare Ferenczi to Freud, April 17, 1910.

192. Freud, "Recommendations to Physicians Practising Psycho-Analysis" (1912), in *SE* 12: 118.

193. See Freud, "Transference-Love," p. 164.

194. Freud, "The Future Prospects of Psycho-Analytic Therapy," p. 145.

195. Freud, "Recommendations to Physicians Practising Psycho-Analysis," p. 116.

196. Freud, "On Beginning the Treatment," p. 126.

197. Freud, "Analysis Terminable and Interminable," pp. 248, 249.

198. Freud, "The Disposition to Obsessional Neurosis: A Contribution to the Problem of Choice of Neurosis" (1913), in *SE* 12: 320.

199. Freud, *The Interpretation of Dreams,* p. 216 (emphasis in the original). Compare Ferenczi to Freud, October 27, 1914.

200. Freud, "Recommendations to Physicians Practising Psycho-Analysis," pp. 111–112, 115; see also Freud, "Two Encyclopaedia Articles" (1923), in *SE* 18: 239.

201. Note the following report: "I have, interestingly enough, tracked down a symptomatic action in myself. While I am analysing and am waiting for the patient's reply, I often cast a quick glance at the picture of my parents. I know now that I always do this when I am following up the patient's infantile transference. The glance is always accompanied by a certain guilt feeling: what will they think of me? This is of course connected with my breaking away from them, which was not easy. Since explaining this symptomatic action to myself, I have not caught myself at it any more." Abraham to Freud, April 7, 1909, *F/A Letters,* p. 77.

Conclusion: Let the Exploration Continue

1. William James, *The Works of William James: Manuscript Lectures* (Cambridge, Mass.: Harvard University Press, 1988), p. 29.

2. Freud, "The Unconscious" (1915), in *SE* 14: 168.

3. Josef Breuer and Sigmund Freud, *Studies on Hysteria* (1893–1895), in *SE* 2: 92.

4. Freud, "Notes upon a Case of Obsessional Neurosis" (1909), in *SE* 10: 157.

5. Freud, "Instincts and Their Vicissitudes" (1915), in *SE* 14: 122.

6. Freud, *The Ego and the Id* (1923), in *SE* 19: 26.

7. Freud, "The Analysis of a Phobia in a Five-Year-Old Boy" (1909), in *SE* 10: 7, 22, 37, 41, 135 (emphasis in the original).

8. Daniel Paul Schreber, *Memoirs of My Nervous Illness,* trans. and ed. by Ida Macalpine and Richard A. Hunter (Cambridge, Mass.: Harvard University Press, 1988), p. 205.

9. Freud, *The Interpretation of Dreams* (1900), in *SE* 4: 173.

10. Freud, "From the History of an Infantile Neurosis" (1918), in *SE* 17: 97.

11. Freud, *Leonardo da Vinci and a Memory of His Childhood* (1910), in *SE* 11: 100 (emphasis in the original).

12. Ibid., p. 117.
13. See Peter Gay, *Freud: A Life for Our Time* (New York: Norton, 1988), pp. 290*n*, 333.
14. Freud, "Five Lectures on Psycho-Analysis" (1910), in *SE* 11: 51.
15. Freud, "Remembering, Repeating and Working-Through (Further Recommendations on the Technique of Psycho-Analysis II)" (1914), in *SE* 12: 154.

Selected Bibliography

The following bibliography is limited to commentary helpful for thinking through Freud's project and to items directly pertinent to this study.

Abraham, Karl. *Selected Papers of Karl Abraham*. Translated by Douglas Bryan and Alix Strachey. London: Hogarth Press, 1927. Reprint. London: H. Karnac, Maresfield Reprints, 1979.

Abraham, Nicolas, and Maria Tarok. *The Wolf Man's Magic Word: A Cryptonymy*. Translated by Nicholas Rand. Minneapolis: University of Minnesota Press, 1986.

Aguayo, Joseph. "Charcot and Freud: Some Implications of Late 19th Century French Psychiatry and Politics for the Origins of Psychoanalysis." *Psychoanalysis and Contemporary Thought* 9 (1986): 223–260.

Amacher, Peter. *Freud's Neurological Education and Its Influence on Psychoanalytic Theory*. Psychological Issues, Monograph 16. New York: International Universities Press, 1965.

———— "The Concepts of the Pleasure Principle and Infantile Erogenous Zones Shaped by Freud's Neurological Education." *The Psychoanalytic Quarterly* 43 (1974): 341–362.

Andersson, Ola. *Studies in the Prehistory of Psychoanalysis: The Etiology of Psychoneuroses and Some Related Themes in Sigmund Freud's Scientific Writings and Letters 1886–1896*. Norstedts: Svenska Bokförlaget, 1962.

———— Letter to Dr. Kurt R. Eissler, April 16, 1962. Freud Archives/B24, Library of Congress.

———— "A Supplement to Freud's Case of 'Frau Emmy von N.' in Studies on Hysteria 1895." *Scandinavian Psychoanalytic Review* 2 (1979): 5–16.

Andreas-Salomé, Lou. *The Freud Journal of Lou Andreas-Salomé*. Translated by Stanley A. Leavy. New York: Basic Books, 1964.

Anzieu, Didier. *Freud's Self-Analysis*. Translated by Peter Graham. London: Hogarth Press, 1986.

—— "The Place of Germanic Language and Culture in Freud's Discovery of Psychoanalysis Between 1895 and 1900." *IJP* 67 (1986): 219–226.

Appignanesi, Lisa, and John Forrester. *Freud's Women.* New York: Basic Books, 1992.

Apfelbaum, Bernard. "On Ego Psychology: A Critique of the Structural Approach to Psycho-Analytic Theory." *IJP* 47 (1966): 451–475.

Ayer, A. J. *The Origins of Pragmatism: Studies in the Philosophy of Charles Sanders Peirce and William James.* San Francisco: Freeman, Cooper, 1968.

Balmary, Marie. *Psychoanalyzing Psychoanalysis: Freud and the Hidden Fault of the Father.* Translated by Ned Lukacher. Baltimore: Johns Hopkins University Press, 1982.

Barclay, James R. "Franz Brentano and Sigmund Freud." *Journal of Existentialism* 5 (1964): 1–36.

Baumeyer, Franz. "The Schreber Case." *IJP* 37 (1956): 61–74.

Beigler, Jerome S. "A Commentary on Freud's Treatment of the Rat Man." *Annual of Psychoanalysis* 3 (1975): 271–285.

Bernfeld, Siegfried. "Freud's Earliest Theories and the School of Helmholtz." *The Psychoanalytic Quarterly* 13 (1944): 341–362.

—— "An Unknown Autobiographical Fragment by Freud." *American Imago* 4 (1946–1947): 3–19.

—— "Freud's Scientific Beginnings." *American Imago* 6 (1949) 163–196.

—— "Sigmund Freud, M. D. 1882–1885." *IJP* 32 (1951): 204–217.

Bernfeld, Siegfried, and Suzanne Cassirer-Bernfeld. "Freud's First Year in Practice, 1886–1887." *Bulletin of the Menninger Clinic* 16 (1952): 37–49.

Bernfeld, Suzanne Cassirer. "Freud and Archaeology." *American Imago* 8 (1951): 107–128.

—— "Discussion of Buxbaum, 'Freud's Dream Interpretation in the Light of His Letters to Fliess.'" *Bulletin of the Menninger Clinic* 16 (1952): 70–72.

Bettelheim, Bruno. *Freud and Man's Soul.* New York: Knopf, 1982.

Bibring, Edward. "The Development and Problems of the Theory of the Instincts." *IJP* 22 (1941): 102–131.

Bird, Brian. "Notes on Transference: Universal Phenomenon and Hardest Part of Analysis." *JAPA* 20 (1972): 267–301.

Bjork, Daniel W. *The Compromised Scientist: William James in the Development of American Psychology.* New York: Columbia University Press, 1983.

Blacker, K. H., and Ruth Abraham. "The Rat Man Revisited: Comments on Maternal Influences." *The International Journal of Psychoanalytic Psychotherapy* 9 (1982): 705–727.

Blanton, Smiley. *Diary of My Analysis with Sigmund Freud.* New York: Hawthorn, 1971.

Blum, Harold P. "On the Conception and Development of the Transference Neurosis." *JAPA* 19 (1971): 41–53.

—— "The Changing Use of Dreams in Psychoanalytic Practice." *IJP* 57 (1976): 315–324.

—— "The Borderline Childhood of the Wolf Man." In *Freud and His Patients*, edited by Mark Kanzer and Jules Glenn. New York: Jason Aronson, 1980.

Boor, Clemens de, and Emma Moersch. "Emmy von N.—eine Hysterie?" *Psyche* 34 (1980): 265–279.

Borch-Jacobsen, Mikkel. *The Freudian Subject*. Translated by Catherine Porter. Stanford, Calif.: Stanford University Press, 1988.

Breger, Louis. *Freud's Unfinished Journey*. London: Routledge and Kegan Paul, 1981.

Brentano, Franz. *Psychology from an Empirical Standpoint*. Translated by Antos C. Rancurello, D. B. Terrell, and Linda McAlister. New York: Humanities Press, 1973.

Breuer, Josef, and Sigmund Freud. "On the Psychical Mechanism of Hysterical Phenomena: Preliminary Communication" (1893). In *SE*, vol. 2.

—— *Studies on Hysteria* (1893–1895). In *SE*, vol. 2.

Brome, Vincent. *Freud and His Early Circle: The Struggles of Psycho-Analysis*. London: Heinemann, 1967.

Brooks, Peter. *Reading for the Plot: Design and Intention in Narrative*. New York: Knopf, 1984.

Brown, Theodore M. "Descartes, Dualism, and Psychosomatic Medicine." In *The Anatomy of Madness: Essays in the History of Psychiatry*. Vol. 1, *People and Ideas*, edited by W. F. Bynum, Roy Porter, and Michael Shepherd. London: Tavistock Publications, 1985.

Browning, Don S. *Pluralism and Personality: William James and Some Contemporary Cultures of Psychology*. Lewisburg, Pa.: Bucknell University Press, 1980.

Bry, Ilse, and Alfred H. Rifkin. "Freud and the History of Ideas: Primary Sources, 1886–1910." In *Psychoanalytic Education*. vol. 5: *Science and Psychoanalysis*, edited by J. Masserman. New York: Grune and Stratton, 1962.

Buckley, Peter. "Fifty Years After Freud: Dora, The Rat Man, and the Wolf Man." *American Journal of Psychiatry* 146 (1989): 1394–1403.

Buxbaum, Edith. "Freud's Dream Interpretation in the Light of His Letters to Fliess." *Bulletin of the Menninger Clinic* 15 (1951): 197–212.

Carella, Michael Jerome. "Psychoanalysis and the Mind-Body Problem." *Psychoanalytic Review* 61 (1974): 53–61.

Carotenuto, Aldo. *A Secret Symmetry: Sabina Spielrein Between Jung and Freud*. Translated by Arno Pomerans, John Shipley, and Krishna Winston. New York: Pantheon, 1982.

Carter, K. Codell. "Infantile Hysteria and Infantile Sexuality in Late Nineteenth-Century German-Language Medical Literature." *Medical History* 27 (1983): 186–196.

Cavell, Marcia. "The Subject of Mind." *IJP* 72 (1991): 141–154.

Chabot, C. Barry. *Freud on Schreber: Psychoanalytic Theory and Critical Act.* Amherst, Mass.: University of Massachusetts Press, 1982.

Chodoff, Paul. "A Critique of Freud's Theory of Infantile Sexuality." *American Journal of Psychiatry* 123 (1966): 507–518.

Clark, Ronald W. *Freud: The Man and the Cause.* New York: Random House, 1980.

Collins, Jane, J. Ray Green, Mary Lydon, Mark Sachner, and Eleanor Honig Skoller. "Questioning the Unconscious: The Dora Archive." In *In Dora's Case: Freud—Hysteria—Feminism,* edited by Charles Bernheimer and Claire Kahane. New York: Columbia University Press, 1985.

Cranefield, Paul F. "Josef Breuer's Evaluation of His Contribution to Psycho-Analysis." *IJP* 39 (1958): 319–322.

———— "Freud and the 'School of Helmholtz.'" *Gesnerus* 23 (1966): 35–39.

Darwin, Charles. *The Works of Charles Darwin,* edited by Paul H. Barrett and R. B. Freeman. Vol. 15, *On the Origin of Species;* vol. 23, *The Descent of Man, and Selection in Relation to Sex* (1871); vol. 24, *The Expression of Emotions in Man and Animal* (1872). London: William Pickering, 1986–1989.

———— *The Life and Letters of Charles Darwin.* 3 vols. Edited by Francis Darwin. London: John Murray, 1887.

———— *More Letters of Charles Darwin.* 2 vols. Edited by Francis Darwin and A. C. Seward. London: John Murray, 1903.

———— *The Autobiography of Charles Darwin.* Edited by Nora Barlow. New York: Norton, 1969.

Daston, Lorraine J. "The Theory of Will Versus the Science of Mind." In *The Problematic Science: Psychology in Nineteenth-Century Thought,* edited by William R. Woodward and Mitchell G. Ash. New York: Praeger, 1982.

David-Ménard, Monique. *Hysteria from Freud to Lacan: Body and Language in Psychoanalysis.* Translated by Catherine Porter. Ithaca, N.Y.: Cornell University Press, 1989.

Davison, Charles. Review of *On Aphasia (A Critical Study),* by Sigmund Freud. *The Psychoanalytic Quarterly* 24 (1955): 115–119.

Decker, Hannah S. *Freud in Germany: Revolution and Reaction in Science, 1893–1907.* Psychological Issues, Monograph 41. New York: International Universities Press, 1977.

———— *Freud, Dora, and Vienna 1900.* New York: Free Press, 1991.

Dennett, Daniel C. *Brainstorms: Philosophical Essays on Mind and Psychology.* Montgomery, Vt.: Bradford Books, 1978.

———— *The Intentional Stance.* Cambridge, Mass.: MIT Press, 1987.

———— *Consciousness Explained.* Boston: Little, Brown, 1991.

Deutsch, Felix. "A Footnote to Freud's 'Fragment of an Analysis of a Case of Hysteria.'" In *In Dora's Case: Freud—Hysteria—Feminism,* edited by Charles Bernheimer and Claire Kahane. New York: Columbia University Press, 1985.

Dewhurst, Kenneth. *Hughlings Jackson on Psychiatry.* Oxford: Sandford Publications, 1982.

Dreyfus, Hubert L., and Paul Rabinow. *Michel Foucault: Beyond Structuralism and Hermeneutics.* 2d ed. Chicago: University of Chicago Press, 1983.

Edelheit, H. "Speech and Psychic Structure: The Vocal-Auditory Organization of the Ego." *JAPA* 17 (1969): 381–412.

Edelson, Marshall. *Hypothesis and Evidence in Psychoanalysis.* Chicago: University of Chicago Press, 1984.

———— *Psychoanalysis: A Theory in Crisis.* Chicago: University of Chicago Press, 1988.

Edinger, Dora. *Bertha Pappenheim: Freud's Anna O.* Highland Park, Ill.: Congregation Solel, 1968.

Eissler, Kurt. R. "The Effect of the Structure of the Ego on Psychoanalytic Technique." *JAPA* 1 (1953): 104–143.

Ellenberger, Henri. *The Discovery of the Unconscious: The History and Evolution of Dynamic Psychiatry.* New York: Basic Books, 1970.

———— "The Story of 'Anna O': A Critical Review with New Data." *Journal of the History of the Behavioral Sciences* 8 (1972): 267–279.

———— "L'histoire d'Emmy von N." *Evolution psychiatrique* 42 (1977): 519–540.

Ellman, Steven. J. *Freud's Technique Papers: A Contemporary Perspective.* Northvale, N.J.: Jason Aronson, 1991.

Elms, Alan C. "Freud, Irma, Martha: Sex and Marriage in the 'Dream of Irma's Injection.'" *Psychoanalytic Review* 67 (1980): 83–109.

Engelhardt, H. T. "John Hughlings Jackson and the Mind-Body Problem." *Bulletin of the History of Medicine* 49 (1975): 137–151.

Erdelyi, M. H. *Psychoanalysis: Freud's Cognitive Science.* New York: Freeman, 1985.

Erikson, Erik Homburger. "The Dream Specimen of Psychoanalysis." *JAPA* 2 (1954): 5–56.

———— *Insight and Responsibility: Lectures on the Ethical Implications of Psychoanalytic Insight.* New York: Norton, 1964.

Fairbairn, W. Ronald D. *Psychoanalytic Studies of the Personality.* London: Tavistock Publications and Routledge and Kegan Paul, 1952.

———— "Theoretical and Experimental Aspects of Psycho-Analysis." *The British Journal of Medical Psychology* 25 (1952): 122–127.

———— "Observations on the Nature of Hysterical States." *The British Journal of Medical Psychology* 27 (1954): 105–125.

———— "On the Nature and Aims of Psycho-Analytical Treatment." *IJP* 39 (1958): 374–385.

———— "Considerations Arising Out of the Schreber Case." *The British Journal of Medical Psychology* 29 (1959): 113–127.

Farrell, B. A. *The Standing of Psychoanalysis*. Oxford: Oxford University Press, 1981.

Feinstein, Howard M. *Becoming William James*. Ithaca, N.Y.: Cornell University Press, 1984.

Fenichel, Otto. *The Psychoanalytic Theory of Neurosis*. New York: Norton, 1945.

Ferenczi, Sándor. Review of *Technik der Psychoanalyse: I. Die analytische Situation*, by Otto Rank. *IJP* 8 (1927): 93–100.

———. *First Contributions to Psycho-Analysis*, 2d ed., translated by Ernst Jones. London: Hogarth Press, 1950.

——— *Further Contributions to the Theory and Technique of Psycho-Analysis* 2d ed., compiled by John Rickman and translated by Jane Isabel Suttie. London: Hogarth Press, 1950.

——— *The Clinical Diary of Sándor Ferenczi*. Edited by Judith Dupont. Translated by Michael Balint and Nicola Zarday Jackson. Cambridge, Mass.: Harvard University Press, 1988.

Ferenczi, Sándor, and Otto Rank. *The Development of Psychoanalysis*. Authorized English ed. by Caroline Newton. Classics in Psychoanalysis, Monograph 4. New York: Nervous and Mental Disease Publishing Co., 1935. Reprint, Madison, Conn.: International Universities Press, 1986.

Fichtner, Gerhard, and Albrecht Hirschmüller. "Freuds 'Katharina'—Hintergrund, Entstehungsgeschichte und Bedeutung einer frühen psychoanalytischen Krankengeschichte." *Psyche* 39 (1985): 220–240.

Fliess, Wilhelm. *Die Beziehungen zwischen Nase und weiblichen Geschlechtsorganen: In ihrer biologischen Bedeutung dargestellt*. Leipzig and Vienna: Franz Deuticke, 1897.

——— *Der Ablauf des Lebens: Grundlegung zur exakten Biologie*. Leipzig and Vienna: Franz Deuticke, 1906.

Forrester, John. *Language and the Origins of Psychoanalysis*. London: Macmillan, 1980.

——— *The Seductions of Psychoanalysis: Freud, Lacan and Derrida*. Cambridge: Cambridge University Press, 1990.

Foucault, Michel. *Madness and Civilization: A History of Insanity in the Age of Reason*. Translated by Richard Howard. New York: Pantheon, 1965.

——— *The Order of Things: An Archaeology of the Human Sciences*. Translated by Alan Sheridan. New York: Pantheon, 1970.

——— *The Archaeology of Knowledge*. Translated by A. M. Sheridan. New York: Pantheon, 1972.

——— *The Birth of the Clinic: An Archaeology of Medical Perception*. Translated by A. M. Sheridan Smith. New York: Pantheon, 1973.

——— *Mental Illness and Psychology*. Translated by Alan Sheridan. New York: Harper and Row, 1976.

——— *Discipline and Punish: The Birth of the Prison*. Translated by Alan Sheridan. New York: Pantheon, 1977.

—— *The History of Sexuality*. Vol 1, *An Introduction*. Translated by Robert Hurley. New York: Pantheon, 1978.

Frampton, Michael F. "Considerations on the Role of Brentano's Concept of Intentionality in Freud's Repudiation of the Seduction Theory." *IRP* 18 (1991): 27–36.

Francher, Raymond E. *Psychoanalytic Psychology: The Development of Freud's Thought*. New York: Norton, 1973.

—— "Brentano's *Psychology from an Empirical Standpoint* and Freud's Early Metapsychology." *Journal of the History of the Behavioral Sciences* 13 (1977): 207–227.

Frankiel, Rita V. "A Note on Freud's Inattention to the Negative Oedipal in Little Hans." *IRP* 18 (1991): 181–184.

—— "Analysed and Unanalysed Themes in the Treatment of Little Hans." *IRP* 19 (1992): 323–333.

Freeman, Lucy. *The Story of Anna O.* New York: Walker, 1972.

Freud, Sigmund. *Gesammelte Werke, chronologisch geordnet*. Edited by Anna Freud, Edward Bibring, Willi Hoffer, Ernst Kris, and Otto Isakower. Vols. 1–17. London: Imago Publishing Co., 1940–1952. Vol. 18. Frankfurt: S. Fischer, 1968.

—— *The Standard Edition of the Complete Psychological Works of Sigmund Freud*. 24 vols. Translated from the German under the general editorship of James Strachey. London: Hogarth Press, 1953–1974.

—— *On Aphasia: A Critical Study* (1891). Translated by E. Stengel. New York: International Universities Press, 1953.

—— *The Origins of Psychoanalysis, Letters to Wilhelm Fliess, Drafts and Notes: 1887–1902*. Edited by Marie Bonaparte, Anna Freud, and Ernst Kris. Translated by Eric Mosbacher and James Strachey. New York: Basic Books, 1954.

—— *Psychoanalysis and Faith: The Letters of Sigmund Freud and Oskar Pfister*. Edited by Heinrich Meng and Ernst L. Freud. Translated by Eric Mosbacher. New York: Basic Books, 1963.

—— *A Psycho-Analytic Dialogue: The Letters of Sigmund Freud and Karl Abraham 1907–1926*. Edited by Hilda C. Abraham and Ernst L. Freud. Translated by Bernard Marsh and Hilda C. Abraham. New York: Basic Books, 1965.

—— *Letters of Sigmund Freud 1873–1939*. Edited by Ernst L. Freud. Translated by Tania Stern and James Stern. London: Hogarth Press, 1970.

—— *The Letters of Sigmund Freud and Arnold Zweig*. Edited by Ernst L. Freud. Translated by Elaine and William Robson-Scott. New York: New York University Press, 1970.

—— *Sigmund Freud and Lou Andreas-Salomé: Letters*. Edited by Ernst Pfeiffer. Translated by Elaine and William Robson-Scott. London: Hogarth Press, 1970.

—— *The Freud/Jung Letters: The Correspondence between Sigmund Freud and*

C. G. Jung. Edited by William McGuire. Translated by Ralph Manheim and R. F. C. Hull. Princeton, N.J.: Princeton University Press, 1974.

———— *L'Homme aux rats: Journal d'une analyse*. Translated by Elza Riberio Hawalka. Paris: Presses Universitaires de France, 1974.

———— *The Complete Letters of Sigmund Freud to Wilhelm Fliess 1887–1904*. Translated and edited by Jeffrey Moussaieff Masson. Cambridge, Mass.: Harvard University Press, 1985.

———— *Sigmund Freud: Briefe an Wilhelm Fliess 1887–1904*. Edited by Jeffrey Moussaieff Masson, assisted by Michael Schröter and Gerhard Fichtner. Frankfurt: S. Fischer, 1986.

———— *A Phylogenetic Fantasy: An Overview of the Transference Neuroses*. Edited by Ilse Grubrich-Simitis. Translated by Axel Hoffer and Peter T. Hoffer. Cambridge, Mass.: Harvard University Press, 1987.

———— *The Letters of Sigmund Freud to Eduard Silberstein 1871–1881*. Edited by Walter Boehlich. Translated by Arnold J. Pomerans. Cambridge, Mass.: Harvard University Press, 1990.

———— Freud-Ferenczi Correspondence. Freud Museum, London.

Friedman, John, and James Alexander. "Psychoanalysis and Natural Science: Freud's 1895 Project Revisited." *IRP* 10 (1983): 303–318.

Fullinwider, S. P. "Sigmund Freud, John Hughlings Jackson, and Speech." *Journal of the History of Ideas* 44 (1983): 151–158.

Galdston, Iago. "Freud and Romantic Medicine." *Bulletin of the History of Medicine* 30 (1956): 489–507.

Gardiner, Muriel, ed. *The Wolf-Man by the Wolf-Man*. New York: Basic Books, 1971.

Garrison, Marsha. "A New Look at Little Hans." *Psychoanalytic Review* 65 (1978): 523–532.

Gauld, Alan. *The Founders of Psychical Research*. New York: Schocken, 1968.

Gay, Peter. *Freud, Jews, and Other Germans: Masters and Victims in Modernist Culture*. New York: Oxford University Press, 1978.

———— *A Godless Jew: Freud, Atheism, and the Making of Psychoanalysis*. New Haven: Yale University Press, 1987.

———— *Freud: A Life for Our Time*. New York: Norton, 1988.

———— *Reading Freud: Explorations and Entertainments*. New Haven: Yale University Press, 1990.

Gedo, John E. *Beyond Interpretation: Toward a Revised Theory for Psychoanalysis*. New York: International Universities Press, 1979.

Gedo, John E., and Arnold Goldberg. *Models of the Mind: A Psychoanalytic Theory*. Chicago: University of Chicago Press, 1973.

Gedo, John E., Melvin Shabshin, Leo Sadow, and Nathan Schlessinger. "*Studies on Hysteria*: A Methodological Evaluation." In *Freud: The Fusion of Science and Humanism: The Intellectual History of Psychoanalysis,* edited by John E. Gedo and George H. Pollock. Psychological Issues, Monograph 34/35. New York: International Universities Press, 1976.

Geha, Richard E. "Freud as Fictionalist: The Imaginary Worlds of Psychoanalysis." In *Freud Appraisals and Reappraisals: Contributions to Freud Studies,* edited by Paul E. Stepansky, vol. 2. Hillsdale, N.J.: Analytic Press, 1988.

Gellner, Ernst. *The Psychoanalytic Movement or The Coming of Unreason.* London: Paladin, 1985.

Gill, Merton M. *Topography and Systems in Psychoanalytic Theory.* Psychological Issues, Monograph 10. New York: International Universities Press, 1963.

———— "The Analysis of the Transference." *JAPA* 27 (suppl.) (1979): 263–288.

———— *Analysis of Transference.* Vol. 1, *Theory and Technique.* Psychological Issues, Monograph 53. New York: International Universities Press, 1982.

Gilson, Lucie. "Franz Brentano on Science and Philosophy." In *The Philosophy of Franz Brentano,* edited by Linda L. McAlister. London: George Duckworth, 1976.

Ginzburg, Carlo. "Morelli, Freud and Sherlock Holmes." *History Workshop* 9 (1980): 5–36.

Glenn, Jules. "Freud's Adolescent Patients: Katharina, Dora, and the 'Homosexual Woman.'" In *Freud and His Patients,* edited by Mark Kanzer and Jules Glenn. New York: Jason Aronson, 1980.

———— "Freud's Advice to Hans's Father: The First Supervisory Sessions." In *Freud and His Patients,* edited by Mark Kanzer and Jules Glenn. New York: Jason Aronson, 1980.

———— "Notes on Psychoanalytic Concepts and Style in Freud's Case Histories." In *Freud and His Patients,* edited by Mark Kanzer and Jules Glenn. New York: Jason Aronson, 1980.

———— "Freud, Dora, and the Maid—A Study of Countertransference." *JAPA* 34 (1986): 591–606.

Glover, Edward. "The Therapeutic Effect of Inexact Interpretation: A Contribution to the Theory of Suggestion." *IJP* 12 (1931): 397–411.

———— *The Technique of Psycho-Analysis.* New York: International Universities Press, 1955.

Glymour, Clark. "The Theory of Your Dreams." In *Physics, Philosophy and Psychoanalysis: Essays in Honor of Adolf Grünbaum.* Boston Studies in the Philosophy of Science no. 76, edited by R. S. Cohen and L. Laudan. Dordrecht, Holland: D. Reidel Publishing Co., 1983.

Graf, Max. "Reminiscences of Professor Freud." *The Psychoanalytic Quarterly* 11 (1942): 465–476.

Greenblatt, S. H. "The Major Influences on the Early Life and Work of John Hughlings Jackson." *Bulletin of the History of Medicine* 39 (1965): 346–376.

———— "Hughlings Jackson's First Encounter with the Work of Paul Broca: The Physiological and Philosophical Background." *Bulletin of the History of Medicine* 44 (1970): 555–570.

Greenberg, R., and C. Pearlman. "If Only Freud Knew: A Reconsideration of Psychoanalytic Dream Theory." *IRP* 5 (1978): 71–75.

Greenson, Ralph R. *The Technique and Practice of Psychoanalysis.* Vol. 1. New York: International Universities Press, 1967.

Gregory, Frederick. *Scientific Materialism in Nineteenth Century Germany.* Dordrecht, Holland: D. Reidel Publishing Co., 1977.

Grigg, Kenneth A. "'All Roads Lead to Rome': The Role of the Nursemaid in Freud's Dreams." *JAPA* 21 (1973): 108–126.

Grinstein, Alexander. *On Sigmund Freud's Dreams.* Detroit, Mich.: Wayne State University Press, 1968.

———— *Freud's Rules of Dream Interpretation.* New York: International Universities Press, 1983.

———— *Freud at the Crossroads.* Madison, Conn.: International Universities Press, 1990.

Groddeck, Georg W. *The Book of the It.* Translated by V. M. E. Collins. London: Vision Press, 1949.

Grosskurth, Phyllis. *The Secret Ring: Freud's Inner Circle and the Politics of Psychoanalysis.* Reading, Mass.: Addison-Wesley, 1991.

Gruber, Howard E. *Darwin on Man: A Psychological Study of Scientific Creativity.* Together with *Darwin's Early and Unpublished Notebooks.* Transcribed and annotated by Paul H. Barrett. New York: E. P. Dutton, 1974.

Grubich-Simitis, Ilse. "Six Letters of Sigmund Freud and Sándor Ferenczi on the Interrelationship of Psychoanalytic Theory and Technique." *IJP* 13 (1986): 259–277.

Grünbaum, Adolf. *The Foundations of Psychoanalysis: A Philosophical Critique.* Berkeley: University of California Press, 1984.

Grunberger, Béla. "Some Reflections on the Rat Man." *IJP* 47 (1966): 160–167.

Gutting, Gary. *Michel Foucault's Archaeology of Scientific Reason.* Cambridge: Cambridge University Press, 1989.

Hale, Nathan G. Jr. *Freud in America,* Vol. 1, *Freud and the Americans: The Beginnings of Psychoanalysis in the United States, 1876–1917.* New York: Oxford University Press, 1971.

———— ed. *James Jackson Putnam and Psychoanalysis: Letters between Putnam and Sigmund Freud, Ernest Jones, William James, Sándor Ferenczi, and Morton Prince, 1877–1917.* Cambridge, Mass.: Harvard University Press, 1971.

Harrington, Anne. *Medicine, Mind, and the Double Brain: A Study in Nineteenth-Century Thought.* Princeton, N.J.: Princeton University Press, 1987.

———— "Hysteria, Hypnosis, and the Lure of the Invisible: The Rise of Neo-mesmerism in *fin-de-siècle* French Psychiatry." In *The Anatomy of Madness.* Vol. 3, *The Asylum and Its Psychiatry,* edited by W. F. Bynum, Roy Porter, and Michael Shepherd. London: Routledge, 1988.

Harris, Adrienne. "Gender as Contradiction." *Psychoanalytic Dialogues* 1 (1991): 197–224.

Hartman, Frank R. "A Reappraisal of the Emma Episode and the Specimen Dream." *JAPA* 31 (1983): 555–585.

Hartmann, Heinz. *Ego Psychology and the Problem of Adaptation* (1939). Translated by David Rapaport. New York: International Universities, Press, 1958.
——— *Essays on Ego Psychology: Selected Problems in Psychoanalytic Theory*. New York: International Universities Press, 1964.
Haynal, André. *The Technique at Issue: Controversies in Psychoanalysis from Freud and Ferenczi to Michael Balint*. Translated by Elizabeth Holder. London: H. Karnac, 1988.
Herbert, Sandra. "The Place of Man in the Development of Darwin's Theory of Transmutation: Part I to July 1837." *Journal of the History of Biology* 7 (1974): 217–258.
——— "The Place of Man in the Development of Darwin's Theory of Transmutation: Part II." *Journal of the History of Biology* 10 (1977): 155–227.
Hertz, Neil. "Dora's Secrets, Freud's Techniques." In *In Dora's Case: Freud—Hysteria—Feminism,* edited by Charles Bernheimer and Claire Kahane. New York: Columbia University Press, 1985.
Herzog, Patricia S. "The Myth of Freud as Anti-Philosopher." In *Freud Appraisals and Reappraisals: Contributions to Freud Studies,* edited by Paul E. Stepansky, vol. 5. Hillsdale, N.J. Analytic Press, 1988.
——— *Conscious and Unconscious: Freud's Dynamic Distinction Reconsidered*. Psychological Issues, Monograph 58. Madison, Conn.: International Universities Press, 1991.
Heimann, Paula. "On Counter-Transference." *IJP* 31 (1950): 81–84.
——— "Problems of the Training Analysis." *IJP* 35 (1954): 163–168.
——— "Dynamics of Transference Interpretations." *IJP* 37 (1956): 303–310.
Hinshelwood, R. D. "Little Hans's Transference." *Journal of Child Psychotherapy* 15 (1989): 63–78.
Hirschmüller, Albrecht. *The Life and Work of Josef Breuer: Physiology and Psychoanalysis*. New York: New York University Press, 1989.
Hoffer, Axel. "The Freud-Ferenczi Controversy: A Living Legacy." *IRP* 18 (1991): 465–472.
Holland, Norman N. "An Identity for the Rat Man." *IRP* 2 (1975): 157–169.
Hollender, Marc H. "The Case of Anna O.: A Reformulation." *American Journal of Psychiatry* 137 (1980): 797–800.
Holt, Robert R. *Freud Reappraised: A Fresh Look at Psychoanalytic Theory*. New York: Guilford Press, 1989.
Hook, Sidney, ed. *Psychoanalysis, Scientific Method, and Philosophy*. New York: New York University Press, 1959.
Hoopes, James. *Consciousness in New England: From Puritanism and Ideas to Psychoanalysis and Semiotic*. Baltimore: Johns Hopkins University Press, 1989.
Hughes, H. Stuart. *Consciousness and Society: The Reorientation of European Social Thought 1890–1930*. New York: Knopf, 1958.
Hughes, Judith M. *Reshaping the Psychoanalytic Domain: The Work of Melanie*

Klein, W. R. D. Fairbairn, and D. W. Winnicott. Berkeley: University of California Press, 1989.

——— "Psychoanalysis as a General Psychology, Revisited." *Free Associations* No. 23 (1991): 357–370.

Hunter, Dianne. "Hysteria, Psychoanalysis, and Feminism: The Case of Anna O." *Feminist Studies* 9 (1983): 465–488.

Hurst, Lindsay C. "What Was Wrong with Anna O.?" *Journal of the Royal Society of Medicine* 75 (1982): 129–131.

——— "Freud and the Great Neurosis: Discussion Paper." *Journal of the Royal Society of Medicine* 76 (1983): 57–61.

Ibsen, Henrik. *Little Eyolf* (1894). Translated by Michael Meyer. London: Methuen, 1980.

Isaacs, Susan. "The Nature and Function of Phantasy." In *Developments in Psycho-Analysis*, Melanie Klein, Paula Heimann, Susan Isaacs and Joan Riviere. London: Hogarth Press, 1952.

Isbister, J. N. *Freud: An Introduction to His Life and Work.* Cambridge: Polity Press, 1985.

Israëls, Han. *Schreber: Father and Son.* Translated by H. S. Lake. Madison, Conn.: International Universities Press, 1989.

Jackson, John Hughlings. "On Affections of Speech from Diseases of the Brain" (1878–1880). In *Selected Writings of John Hughlings Jackson,* edited by James Taylor, vol. 2. New York: Basic Books, 1958.

Jackson, Stanley W. "The History of Freud's Concept of Regression." *JAPA* 17 (1969): 743–784.

Jacobsen, P. B., and R. S. Steele. "From Present to Past: Freudian Archaeology." *IRP* 6 (1979): 349–362.

James, William. *The Works of William James,* under the general editorship of Frederick Burkhardt: *Essays in Psychology; The Principles of Psychology* (3 vols.); *The Varieties of Religious Experience; Essays in Psychical Research; Manuscript Lectures.* Cambridge, Mass.: Harvard University Press, 1979–1988.

——— *The Letters of William James,* edited by Henry James. 2 vols. Boston: Atlantic Monthly Press, 1920.

Janet, Pierre. *L'Automatisme psychologique.* Paris: Félix Alcan, 1889.

Janik, Allan, and Stephen Toulmin. *Wittgenstein's Vienna.* New York: Simon and Schuster, 1973.

Jennings, Jerry L. "The Revival of 'Dora': Advances in Psychoanalytic Theory and Technique." *JAPA* 34 (1986): 607–635.

Jensen, Ellen. "Anna O.: A Study of Her Later Life." *The Psychoanalytic Quarterly* 39 (1970): 269–293.

Jensen, Wilhelm. *Gradiva: Ein pompejanisches Phantasiestück.* Dresden and Leipzig: Carl Reissner, 1903.

——— "Drei unveröffentlichte Briefe von Wilhelm Jensen." *Psychoanalytische Bewegung* 1 (1929): 207–211.

Johnson, Michael G., and Tracy B. Henley, eds. *Reflections on "The Principles of Psychology": William James After a Century*. Hillsdale, N.J.: Lawrence Erlbaum, 1990.

Johnston, William M. *The Austrian Mind: An Intellectual and Social History 1848–1938*. Berkeley: University of California Press, 1972.

Jones, Ernest. "The Origin and Structure of the Super-Ego." *IJP* 7 (1926): 303–311.

—— *The Life and Work of Sigmund Freud*. Vol. 1, *The Formative Years and the Great Discoveries 1856–1900*. Vol. 2, *Years of Maturity 1901–1919*. Vol. 3, *The Last Phase 1919–1939*. New York: Basic Books, 1953–1957.

—— "Freud's Early Travels." *IJP* 35 (1954): 81–84.

—— *Free Associations: Memories of a Psycho-Analyst*. New York: Basic Books, 1959.

—— *Papers on Psycho-Analysis*, 5th ed., by Ernest Jones. London: Ballière, Tindall and Cox, 1948. Reprint, London: H. Karnac, Maresfield Reprints, 1977.

Kanzer, Mark. Review of *The Wolf-Man by the Wolf-Man*, edited by Muriel Gardner. *IJP* 53 (1972): 419–422.

—— "Two Prevalent Misconceptions about Freud's Project (1895)." *Annual of Psychoanalysis* 1 (1973): 88–103.

—— "Freud's 'Human Influence' on the Rat Man." In *Freud and His Patients*, edited by Mark Kanzer and Jules Glenn. New York: Jason Aronson, 1980.

—— "Further Comments on the Wolf Man: The Search for the Primal Scene." In *Freud and His Patients*, edited by Mark Kanzer and Jules Glenn. New York: Jason Aronson, 1980.

—— "The Transference Neurosis of the Rat Man." In *Freud and His Patients*, edited by Mark Kanzer and Jules Glenn. New York: Jason Aronson, 1980.

Kanzer, Mark, and Jules Glenn, eds. *Freud and His Self-Analysis*. New York: Jason Aronson, 1979.

Kaplan, Marion. *The Jewish Feminist Movement in Germany: The Campaign of the Jüdischer Frauenbund, 1904–1938*. Westport, Conn.: Greenwood, 1979.

Kardiner, Abram. *My Analysis with Freud: Reminiscences*. New York: Norton, 1977.

Karpe, Richard. "The Rescue Complex in Anna O.'s Final Identity." *The Psychoanalytic Quarterly* 30 (1961): 1–24.

Keill, Norman. *Freud without Hindsight: Reviews of His Work (1893–1939) By His Contemporaries*. Madison, Conn.: International Universities Press, 1988.

Kermode, Frank. "Freud and Interpretation." *IRP* 12 (1985): 3–12.

Kern, Stephen. "Freud and the Discovery of Child Sexuality." *History of Childhood Quarterly: The Journal of Psychohistory* 1 (1973): 117–141.

—— *Anatomy and Destiny: A Cultural History of the Human Body*. Indianapolis and New York: Bobbs-Merrill, 1975.

Kerr, John. "Beyond the Pleasure Principle and Back Again: Freud, Jung, and Sabina Spielrein." In *Freud Appraisals and Reappraisals: Contributions to*

Freud Studies, edited by Paul E. Stepansky, vol. 3. Hillsdale, N.J.: Analytic Press, 1988.

Khan, M. Masud R. "The Changing Use of Dreams in Psychoanalytic Practice." *IJP* 57 (1976): 325–330.

Kitcher, Patricia W. *Freud's Dream: A Complete Interdisciplinary Science of Mind.* Cambridge, Mass.: MIT Press, 1992.

Klein, D. B. *A History of Scientific Psychology: Its Origins and Philosophical Backgrounds.* New York: Basic Books, 1970.

Klein, George S. *Psychoanalytic Theory: An Exploration of Essentials.* New York: International Universities Press, 1976.

Knight, Isabel F. "Freud's 'Project': A Theory for *Studies on Hysteria.*" *Journal of the History of the Behavioral Sciences* 20 (1984): 340–358.

Kohon, Gregorio. "Reflections on Dora: The Case of Hysteria." *IJP* 65 (1984): 73–84.

Krafft-Ebing, Richard von. *Psychopathia sexualis, mit besonderer Berücksichtigung der conträren Sexualempfindung. Eine medizinisch-gerichtliche Studie für Ärtze und Juristen.* 12th ed. Stuttgart: F. Enke, 1903. (Translated by Franklin S. Klaf as *Psychopathia Sexualis, with Especial Reference to the Antipathic Sexual Instinct: A Medico-Forensic Study.* New York: Bell, 1965.)

Kravis, Nathan M. "The 'Prehistory' of the Idea of Transference." *IRP* 19 (1992): 9–22.

Kris, Ernst. "Ego Psychology and Interpretation in Psychoanalytic Therapy." *The Psychoanalytic Quarterly* 20 (1951): 15–30.

———— Introduction to *The Origins of Psychoanalysis, Letters to Wilhelm Fliess, Drafts and Notes: 1887–1902,* by Sigmund Freud. Edited by Marie Bonaparte, Anna Freud, and Ernst Kris. Translated by Eric Mosbacher and James Strachey. New York: Basic Books, 1954.

Krohn, Alan. *Hysteria: The Elusive Neurosis.* Psychological Issues, Monograph 45/46. New York: International Universities Press, 1978.

Krüll, Marianne. *Freud and His Father.* Translated by Arnold J. Pomerans. New York: Norton, 1986.

Kuper, Adam, and Alan A. Stone. "The Dream of Irma's Injection: A Structural Analysis." *American Journal of Psychiatry* 139 (1982): 1225–1234.

Langs, Robert. "The Misalliance Dimension in the Case of Dora." In *Freud and His Patients,* edited by Mark Kanzer and Jules Glenn. New York: Jason Aronson, 1980.

———— "The Misalliance Dimension in the Case of the Rat Man." In *Freud and His Patients,* edited by Mark Kanzer and Jules Glenn. New York: Jason Aronson, 1980.

———— "The Misalliance Dimension in the Case of the Wolf Man." In *Freud and His Patients,* edited by Mark Kanzer and Jules Glenn. New York: Jason Aronson, 1980.

———— "Freud's Irma Dream and the Origins of Psychoanalysis." *Psychoanalytic Review* 71 (1984): 591–617.

Laplanche, Jean. *New Foundations for Psychoanalysis.* Translated by David Macey. Oxford: Basil Blackwell, 1989.

Laplanche, Jean, and J.-B. Pontalis. "Fantasy and the Origins of Sexuality." *IJP* 49 (1968): 1–18.

———— *The Language of Psycho-Analysis.* Translated by Donald Nicholson-Smith. London: Hogarth Press, 1980.

Laqueur, Thomas. *Making Sex: Body and Gender from Greeks to Freud.* Cambridge, Mass.: Harvard University Press, 1990.

Leary, David Edward. "The Reconstruction of Psychology in Germany, 1780–1850." Ph.D. dissertation, University of Chicago, 1977.

———— "The Philosophical Conception of Psychology in Germany, 1780–1850." *Journal of the History of the Behavioral Sciences* 14 (1978): 113–121.

———— "Wundt and After: Psychology's Shifting Relations with the Natural Sciences, Social Sciences, and Philosophy." *Journal of the History of the Behavioral Sciences* 15 (1979): 231–241.

Leavitt, Harry C. "A Biological and Teleological Study of 'Irma's Injection' Dream." *Psychoanalytic Review* 43 (1956): 440–447.

Lesky, Erna. *The Vienna Medical School of the Nineteenth Century.* Baltimore: Johns Hopkins University Press, 1976.

Levin, Kenneth. "Freud's Paper 'On Male Hysteria' and the Conflict between Anatomical and Physiological Models." *Bulletin of the History of Medicine* 48 (1974): 377–397.

———— *Freud's Early Psychology of the Neuroses: A Historical Perspective.* Pittsburgh Pa.: University of Pittsburgh Press, 1978.

Lewin, Karl K. "Dora Revisited." *Psychoanalytic Review* 60 (1974): 519–532.

Lewis, Nolan D. C., and Carney Landis. "Freud's Library." *Psychoanalytic Review* 44 (1957): 327–354.

Lieberman, E. James. *Acts of Will: The Life and Work of Otto Rank.* New York: Free Press, 1985.

Linschoten, Hans. *On the Way Toward a Phenomenological Psychology: The Psychology of William James.* Duquesne Studies, Psychological Series, edited by Amedeo Giorgi, no. 5. Pittsburgh, Pa.: Duquesne University Press, 1968.

Lipton, Samuel D. "The Advantages of Freud's Technique as Shown in His Analysis of the Rat Man." *IJP* 58 (1977): 255–273.

———— "An Addendum to 'The Advantages of Freud's Technique as Shown in His Analysis of the Rat Man.'" *IJP* 60 (1979): 215–216.

Loewald, Hans. *Papers on Psychoanalysis.* New Haven: Yale University Press, 1980.

Lothane, Zvi. "Schreber, Freud, Flechsig, and Weber Revisited: An Inquiry into Methods of Interpretation." *Psychoanalytic Review* 76 (1989): 203–262.

MacIntyre, A. C. *The Unconscious: A Conceptual Analysis.* New York: Humanities Press, 1958.

MacKay, Nigel. *Motivation and Explanation: An Essay on Freud's Philosophy of Science.* Madison, Conn.: International Universities Press, 1989.

Macmillan, Malcolm B. "Freud's Expectations and the Childhood Seduction Theory." *Australian Journal of Psychology* 29 (1977): 223–236.

—— "Delboeuf and Janet as Influences in Freud's Treatment of Emmy von N." *Journal of the History of the Behavioral Sciences* 15 (1979): 299–309.

—— "Freud and Janet on Organic and Hysterical Paralyses: A Mystery Solved?" *IRP* 17 (1990): 189–203.

Madison, Peter. *Freud's Concept of Repression and Defense, Its Theoretical and Observational Language.* Minneapolis: University of Minnesota Press, 1961.

Mahony, Patrick J. "Towards a Formalist Approach to Dreams." *IRP* 4 (1977): 83–98.

—— "Friendship and Its Discontents." *Contemporary Psychoanalysis* 15 (1979): 55–109.

—— *Cries of the Wolf Man.* New York: International Universities Press, 1984.

—— *Freud and the Rat Man.* New Haven: Yale University Press, 1986.

—— *Freud as a Writer.* Expanded ed. New Haven: Yale University Press, 1987.

—— *On Defining Freud's Discourse.* New Haven: Yale University Press, 1989.

Major, René. "The Language of Interpretation." *IRP* 1 (1974): 425–435.

Malcolm, Janet. *Psychoanalysis: The Impossible Profession.* New York: Knopf, 1981.

—— *In the Freud Archives.* New York: Knopf, 1984.

Marcus, Steven. *Freud and the Culture of Psychoanalysis: Studies in the Transition from Victorian Humanism to Modernity.* New York: Norton, 1984.

Marty, Pierre, Michel Fain, Michel de M'Uzan, and Christian David. "Der Fall Dora und der psychosomatische Gesichtspunkt." *Psyche* 33 (1979): 888–925.

Masson, Jeffrey Moussaieff. Review of *Gespräche mit dem Wolfsmann: Eine Psychanalyse und die Folgen,* by Karin Obholzer. *IRP* 9 (1982): 116–119.

—— *The Assault on Truth: Freud's Suppression of the Seduction Theory.* New York: Farrar, Straus and Giroux, 1984.

McCaffrey, Phillip. *Freud and Dora: The Artful Dream.* New Brunswick, N.J.: Rutgers University Press, 1984.

McGrath, William J. *Freud's Discovery of Psychoanalysis: The Politics of Hysteria.* Ithaca, N.Y.: Cornell University Press, 1986.

McGuire, Michael T. *Reconstructions in Psychoanalysis.* New York: Appleton, Century, Crofts, 1971.

McIntosh, Donald. "The Ego and the Self in the Thought of Sigmund Freud." *IJP* 67 (1986): 429–449.

Meissner, W. W. "A Note on Internalization as Process." *The Psychoanalytic Quarterly* 45 (1976): 374–393.

—— "Studies on Hysteria—Katharina." *The Psychoanalytic Quarterly* 48 (1979): 587–600.

—— "A Study on Hysteria: Anna O. Rediviva." *Annual of Psychoanalysis* 7 (1979): 17–52.

—— "Studies on Hysteria—Frau von N." *Bulletin of the Menninger Clinic* 45 (1981): 1–19.

Meltzer, Donald. *The Kleinian Development: Part I, Freud's Clinical Development (Method-Data-Therapy).* Perthshire: Clunie Press, 1978.

Meltzer, Françoise, ed. *The Trial(s) of Psychoanalysis.* Chicago: University of Chicago Press, 1988.

Merejkowski, Dimitri. *The Romance of Leonardo da Vinci.* Translated by Bernard Guilbert Guerney. New York: Random House, 1928.

Micale, Mark S. " Hysteria and Its Historiography: A Review of Past and Present Writings (1)." *History of Science* 27 (1989): 223–262.

——— "Hysteria and Its Historiography: A Review of Past and Present Writings (2)." *History of Science* 27 (1989): 319–351.

——— "Hysteria and Its Historiography: The Future Perspective." *History of Psychiatry* 1 (1990): 33–124.

Minutes of the Vienna Psychoanalytic Society. 4 vols. Edited by Herman Nunberg and Ernst Federn. Translated by M. Nunberg. New York: International Universities Press, 1962–1975.

Moi, Toril. "Representation of Patriarchy: Sexuality and Epistemology in Freud's Dora." In *In Dora's Case: Freud—Hysteria—Feminism,* edited by Charles Bernheimer and Claire Kahane. New York: Columbia University Press, 1985.

Moll, Albert. *Perversions of the Sex Instinct: A Study of Sexual Inversion Based on Clinical Data and Official Documents.* Translated by Maurice Popkin. Newark, N.J.: Julian Press, 1931.

——— *Untersuchungen über die Libido sexualis.* Berlin: Fischer's Medizinsche Buchhandlung, 1897. (Translated and abridged by David Berger as *Libido Sexualis: Studies in the Psychosexual Laws of Love Verified by Clinical Sexual Case Histories.* New York: American Ethnological Press, 1933.)

Momigliano, Luciana Nissim. "A Spell in Vienna—But Was Freud a Freudian? An Investigation into Freud's Technique between 1920 and 1938, Based on the Published Testimony of Former Analysands." *IRP* 14 (1987): 373–389.

Muslin, Hyman L. "Transference in the Rat Man Case: The Transference in Transition." *JAPA* 27 (1979): 561–578.

Muslin, Hyman, and Merton Gill. "Transference in the Dora Case." *JAPA* 26 (1978): 311–328.

Myers, Gerald E. *William James: His Life and Thought.* New Haven: Yale University Press, 1986.

Neu, Jerome, ed. *The Cambridge Companion to Freud.* Cambridge: Cambridge University Press, 1991.

Niederland, William G. *The Schreber Case: Psychoanalytic Profile of a Paranoid Personality.* New York: Quadrangle/New York Times, 1974.

Novey, Samuel. *The Second Look: The Reconstruction of Personal History in Psychiatry and Psychoanalysis.* Baltimore: Johns Hopkins University Press, 1968.

Obholzer, Karin. *The Wolf-Man Sixty Years Later: Conversations with Freud's Controversial Patient.* Translated by Michael Shaw. London: Routledge and Kegan Paul, 1982.

Oppenheim, Janet. *The Other World: Spiritualism and Psychical Research in England, 1850–1914.* Cambridge: Cambridge University Press, 1985.

Ornston, Darius Gray Jr. "Strachey's Influence: A Preliminary Report." *IJP* 63 (1982): 409–426.

—— "Freud's Conception Is Different from Strachey's." *JAPA* 33 (1985): 379–412.

—— "The Invention of 'Cathexis' and Strachey's Strategy." *IRP* 12 (1985): 391–399.

—— "How Standard Is the 'Standard Edition'?" In *Freud in Exile: Psychoanalysis and Its Vicissitudes,* edited by Edward Timms and Naomi Segal. New Haven: Yale University Press, 1988.

Orr-Andrawes, Alison. "The Case of Anna O.: A Neuropsychiatric Perspective." *JAPA* 35 (1987): 387–419.

Otto, M. M. "Freud and Aphasia: An Historical Analysis." *American Journal of Psychiatry* 124 (1967): 815–825.

Owen, A. R. *Hysteria, Hypnosis and Healing: The Work of J.-M. Charcot.* London: Dennis Dobson, 1971.

Pankejeff, Sergei. "Letters Pertaining to Freud's 'History of an Infantile Neurosis.'" *The Psychoanalytic Quarterly* 26 (1957): 449–460.

Pappenheim, Else. "Freud and Gilles de la Tourette: Diagnostic Speculations on 'Frau Emmy von N.'" *IRP* 7 (1980): 265–277.

—— "More on the Case of Anna O." *American Journal of Psychiatry* 137 (1980): 1625–1626.

Perry, Ralph Barton. *The Thought and Character of William James.* 2 vols. Boston: Little, Brown, 1935.

Pollock, George H. "The Possible Significance of Childhood Object Loss in the Josef Breuer—Bertha Pappenheim (Anna O.)—Sigmund Freud Relationship. I. Josef Breuer." *JAPA* 16 (1968): 711–739.

—— "Bertha Pappenheim's Pathological Mourning: Possible Effects of Childhood Sibling Loss." *JAPA* 20 (1972): 476–493.

—— "Josef Breuer." In *Freud: The Fusion of Science and Humanism: The Intellectual History of Psychoanalysis,* edited by John E. Gedo and George H. Pollock. Psychological Issues, Monograph 34/35. New York: International Universities Press, 1976.

Pribram, Karl H. "The Neuropsychology of Sigmund Freud." In *Experimental Foundations of Clinical Psychology,* edited by Arthur J. Bachrach. New York: Basic Books, 1962.

—— "Freud's Project: An Open Biologically Based Model for Psychoanalysis." In *Psychoanalysis and Current Biological Thought,* edited by Norman S. Greenfield and William C. Lewis. Madison: University of Wisconsin Press, 1965.

—— "The Foundation of Psychoanalytic Theory: Freud's Neuropsychological

Model." In *Brain and Behavior.* Vol. 4, *Adaption,* edited by Karl H. Pribram. Harmondsworth: Penguin Books, 1969.

Pribram, Karl H., and Merton M. Gill, *Freud's 'Project' Reassessed: Preface to Contemporary Cognitive Theory and Neurophsychology.* New York: Basic Books, 1976.

Racker, H. *Transference and Countertransference.* New York: International Universities Press, 1968.

Ramas, Maria. "Freud's Dora, Dora's Hysteria." In *In Dora's Case: Freud—Hysteria—Feminism,* edited by Charles Bernheimer and Claire Kahane. New York: Columbia University Press, 1985.

Rapaport, David. *The Structure of Psychoanalytic Theory.* Psychological Issues, Monograph 6. New York: International Universities Press, 1960.

Reeves, Christopher. "Breuer, Freud and the Case of Anna O.: A Reexamination." *Journal of Child Psychotherapy* 8 (1982): 203–214.

Richards, Robert J. "Wundt's Early Theories of Unconscious Inference and Cognitive Evolution in Their Relation to Darwinian Biopsychology." In *Wundt Studies,* edited by Wolfgang Bringmann and Ryan D. Tweney. Toronto: Hogrefe, 1980.

———— "Darwin and the Biologizing of Moral Behavior." In *The Problematic Science: Psychology in Nineteenth Century Thought,* edited by William R. Woodward and Mitchell G. Ash. New York: Praeger, 1982.

———— *Darwin and the Emergence of Evolutionary Theories of Mind and Behavior.* Chicago: University of Chicago Press, 1987.

Ricoeur, Paul. *Freud and Philosophy: An Essay on Interpretation.* Translated by Denis Savage. New Haven: Yale University Press, 1970.

———— "The Question of Proof in Freud's Psychoanalytic Writings." *JAPA* 25 (1977): 835–871.

Rieff, Philip. *Freud: The Mind of the Moralist.* New York: Viking Press, 1959.

———— Introduction to *Dora: An Analysis of a Case of Hysteria,* by Sigmund Freud. New York: Collier, 1963.

Riese, Walter. "Freudian Concepts of Brain Function and Brain Disease." *The Journal of Nervous and Mental Diseases* 127 (1958): 287–307.

———— "The Neuropsychologic Phase in the History of Psychiatric Thought." In *Historic Derivations of Modern Psychiatry,* edited by Iago Galdston. New York: McGraw-Hill, 1967.

Ritvo, Lucille B. "Darwin as the Source of Freud's Neo-Lamarckianism." *JAPA* 13 (1965): 499–517.

———— "Carl Claus as Freud's Professor of the New Darwinian Biology." *IJP* 53 (1972): 277–283.

———— "The Impact of Darwin on Freud." *The Psychoanalytic Quarterly* 43 (1974): 177–192.

———— *Darwin's Influence on Freud: A Tale of Two Sciences.* New Haven: Yale University Press, 1990.

Riviere, Joan. "A Contribution to the Analysis of the Negative Therapeutic Reaction." *IJP* 17 (1936): 304–320.

———— "A Character Trait of Freud's." In *Psycho-Analysis and Contemporary Thought,* edited by John D. Sutherland. London: Hogarth Press, 1958.

Rizzuto, Ana-Maria. "A Hypothesis about Freud's Motive for Writing the Monograph 'On Aphasia.'" *IRP* 16 (1989): 111–117.

———— "The Origins of Freud's Concept of Object Representation ('Objektvorstellung') in His Monograph 'On Aphasia': Its Theoretical and Technical Importance." *IJP* 71 (1990): 241–248.

———— "Freud's Theoretical and Technical Models in *Studies on Hysteria.*" *IRP* 19 (1992): 169–177.

Roazen, Paul. *Freud and His Followers.* New York: Knopf, 1975.

Robert, W. *Der Traum als Naturnothwendigkeit erklärt.* Hamburg: Hermann Seippel, 1886.

Robinson, Daniel N. *An Intellectual History of Psychology.* Rev. ed. New York: Macmillan, 1981.

Robinson, Paul. *Freud and His Critics.* Berkeley: University of California Press, 1993.

Rogow, Arnold A. "A Further Footnote to Freud's 'Fragment of an Analysis of a Case of Hysteria.'" *JAPA* 26 (1978): 330–356.

Rose, Jacqueline. "Dora—A Fragment of an Analysis." In *In Dora's Case: Freud—Hysteria—Feminism,* edited by Charles Bernheimer and Claire Kahane. New York: Columbia University Press, 1985.

Rosenbaum, Max, and Melvin Muroff, eds. *Anna O.: Fourteen Contemporary Reinterpretations.* New York: Free Press, 1984.

Rosenblatt, Allan D. "Epilogue: Transference Neurosis: Phenomenon in Search of a Referent." *Psychoanalytic Inquiry* 7 (1987): 599–603.

Rosenfeld, Herbert. "Critical Appreciaton of James Strachey's Paper on 'The Nature of the Therapeutic Action of Psychoanalysis.'" *IJP* 53 (1972): 455–462.

———— "Negative Therapeutic Reaction." In *Tactics and Techniques in Psychoanalytic Therapy.* Vol. 2, *Countertransference,* edited by Peter L. Giovacchini. New York: Jason Aronson, 1975.

Rosenfeld, Israel. *The Invention of Memory: A New View of the Brain.* New York: Basic Books, 1988.

Rosenzweig, Saul. *Freud, Jung, and Hall the King-Maker: The Historic Expedition to America (1909).* Seattle: Hogrefe and Huber, 1992.

Ross, Barbara. "William James: A Prime Mover of the Psychoanalytic Movement in America." In *Psychoanalysis, Psychotherapy, and the New England Medical Scene 1894–1944,* edited by George E. Gifford, Jr. New York: Science History Publications, 1978.

Roudinesco, Elisabeth. *La bataille de cent ans: Histoire de la psychanalyse en France.* Vol. 1, *1885–1939.* Paris: Editions Ramsay, 1982.

Rubinstein, Benjamin B. "Psychoanalytic Theory and the Mind-Body Problem." In *Psychoanalysis and Current Biological Thought,* edited by Norman S. Greenfield and William C. Lewis. Madison: University of Wisconsin Press, 1965.

—— "Freud's Early Theories of Hysteria." In *Physics, Philosophy and Psychoanalysis: Essays in Honor of Adolf Grünbaum.* Boston Studies in the Philosophy of Science no. 76, edited by R. S. Cohen. Dordrecht, Holland: D. Reidel Publishing Co., 1983.

Rudnytsky, Peter L. *Freud and Oedipus.* New York: Columbia University Press, 1987.

Rustin, Michael. "The Social Organization of Secrets: Towards a Sociology of Psychoanalysis." *IRP* 12 (1985): 143–159.

Ryan, Judith. "American Pragmatism, Viennese Psychology." *Raritan* 7 (1989): 45–54.

Rycroft, Charles. *A Critical Dictionary of Psychoanalysis.* New York: Basic Books, 1968.

—— *The Innocence of Dreams.* London: Hogarth Press, 1979.

Sachs, Hanns. *Freud: Master and Friend.* Cambridge, Mass.: Harvard University Press, 1944.

Sandler, Joseph. "Countertransference and Role Responsiveness." *IRP* 3 (1976): 43–47.

—— "Unconscious Wishes and Human Relationships." *Contemporary Psychoanalysis* 17 (1981): 180–196.

—— "Reflections on Some Relations Between Psychoanalytic Concepts and Psychoanalytic Practice." *IJP* 64 (1983): 35–45.

Sandler, Joseph, and Christopher Dare. "The Psychoanalytic Concept of Orality." *Journal of Psychosomatic Research* 14 (1970): 211–222.

Sandler, Joseph, and Humberto Nagera. "Aspects of the Metapsychology of Fantasy." *The Psychoanalytic Study of the Child* 18 (1963): 159–194.

Sandler, Joseph, and Bernard Rosenblatt. "The Concept of the Representational World." *The Psychoanalytic Study of the Child* 17 (1962): 128–145.

Sandler, Joseph, and Anne-Marie Sandler. "The 'Second-Censorship', the 'Three Box Model' and Some Technical Implications." *IJP* 64 (1983): 413–424.

—— "The Past Unconscious, the Present Unconscious, and Interpretation of the Transference." *Psychoanalytic Inquiry* 4 (1984): 367–399.

Schafer, Roy. *Aspects of Internalization.* New York: International Universities Press, 1968.

—— *A New Language for Psychoanalysis.* New Haven: Yale University Press, 1976.

—— *The Analytic Attitude.* New York: Basic Books, 1983.

—— *Retelling a Life.* New York: Basic Books, 1992.

Schatzman, Morton. *Soul Murder: Persecution in the Family.* New York: Random House, 1973.

Scheffler, Israel. *Four Pragmatists: A Critical Introduction to Peirce, James, Mead, and Dewey.* New York: Humanities Press, 1974.

Schiller, Francis. *A Möbius Strip: Fin-de-Siècle Neuropsychiatry and Paul Möbius.* Berkeley: University of California Press, 1982.

Schimek, Jean G. "Fact and Fantasy in the Seduction Theory: A Historical Review." *JAPA* 35 (1987): 937–966.

Schlesinger, Nathan, et al. "The Scientific Styles of Breuer and Freud and the Origins of Psychoanalysis." In *Freud: The Fusion of Science and Humanism: The Intellectual History of Psychoanalysis,* edited by John E. Gedo and George H. Pollock. Psychological Issues, Monograph 34/35. New York: International Universities Press, 1976.

Schneiderman, Stuart. *Rat Man.* New York: New York University Press, 1986.

Schorske, Carl. *Fin-de-Siècle Vienna: Politics and Culture.* New York: Knopf, 1980.

Schreber, Daniel Paul. *Memoirs of My Nervous Illness.* Edited and translated by Ida Macalpine and Richard A. Hunter. Cambridge, Mass.: Harvard University Press, 1988.

Schur, Max. "Some Additional 'Day Residues' of the 'Specimen Dream of Psychoanalysis.'" In *Psychoanalysis—A General Psychology: Essays in Honor of Heniz Hartmann,* edited by R. M. Loewenstein, L. M. Newman, M. Schur, and A. J. Solnit. New York: International Universities Press, 1966.

——— *Freud: Living and Dying.* New York: International Universities Press, 1972.

——— "The Background to Freud's 'Disturbance' on the Acropolis." In *Freud and His Self-Analysis,* edited by Mark Kanzer and Jules Glenn. New York: Jason Aronson, 1979.

Schur, Max, and Lucille B. Ritvo. "The Concept of Development and Evolution in Psychoanalysis." In *Development and Evolution of Behavior: Essays in Memory of T. C. Schneirla,* edited by Lester R. Aronson and Ethel Toback. San Francisco: Freeman, 1970.

Sharpe, Ella Freeman. *Dream Analysis: A Practical Handbook for Psycho-Analysts.* London: Hogarth Press, 1937.

Shengold, Leonard. "More About Rats and Rat People." In *Freud and His Patients,* edited by Mark Kanzer and Jules Glenn. New York: Jason Aronson, 1980.

——— *Soul Murder: The Effects of Childhood Abuse and Deprivation.* New Haven: Yale University Press, 1989.

Sherwood, Michael. *The Logic of Explanation in Psychoanalysis.* New York: Academic Press, 1969.

Shorter, Edward. *From Paralysis to Fatigue: A History of Psychosomatic Illness in the Modern Era.* New York: Free Press, 1992.

Showalter, Elaine. *The Female Malady: Women, Madness, and English Culture, 1830–1980.* New York: Pantheon, 1985.

Silverman, Martin A. "A Fresh Look at the Case of Little Hans." In *Freud and*

His Patients, edited by Mark Kanzer and Jules Glenn. New York: Jason Aronson, 1980.

Silverstein, Barry. "Freud's Psychology and Its Organic Foundation: Sexuality and Mind-Body Interactionism." *Psychoanalytic Review* 72 (1985): 203–228.

——— "Oedipal Politics and Scientific Creativity—Freud's 1915 Phylogenetic Fantasy." *Psychoanalytic Review* 76 (1989): 403–424.

Slipp, Samuel. "Interpersonal Factors in Hysteria: Freud's Seduction Theory and the Case of Dora." *Journal of the American Academy of Psychoanalysis* 5 (1977): 359–376.

Smith, C. U. M. "Evolution and the Problem of Mind. Part II. John Hughlings Jackson." *Journal of the History of Biology* 15 (1982): 241–262.

Solms, Mark, and Michael Saling. "On Psychoanalysis and Neuroscience: Freud's Attitude to the Localizationist Tradition." *IJP* 67 (1986): 397–416.

Spence, Donald P. *Narrative Truth and Historical Truth: Meaning and Interpretation in Psychoanalysis.* New York: Norton, 1982.

——— *The Freudian Metaphor: Toward Paradigm Change in Psychoanalysis.* New York: Norton, 1987.

Sprengether, Madelon. "Enforcing Oedipus: Freud and Dora." In *In Dora's Case: Freud—Hysteria—Feminism,* edited by Charles Bernheimer and Claire Kahane. New York: Columbia University Press, 1985.

——— *The Spectral Mother: Freud, Feminism, and Psychoanalysis.* Ithaca, N. Y.: Cornell University Press, 1990.

Stanton, Martin. *Sándor Ferenczi: Reconsidering Active Intervention.* London: Free Association Books, 1990.

Stein, Martin H. "The Unobjectionable Part of the Transference." *JAPA* 29 (1981): 869–892.

Steiner, Riccardo. "To Explain Our Point of View to English Readers in English Words." *IRP* 18 (1991): 351–392.

Stengel, Erwin. Introduction to *On Aphasia: A Critical Study* by Sigmund Freud. Translated by Erwin Stengel. New York: International Universities Press, 1953.

——— "A Re-Evaluation of Freud's Book 'On Aphasia': Its Significance for Psycho-Analysis." *IJP* 35 (1954): 85–89.

——— "Hughlings Jackson's Influence in Psychiatry." *British Journal of Psychiatry* 109 (1963): 348–355.

Stepansky, Paul E. *In Freud's Shadow: Adler in Context.* Hillsdale, N.J.: Analytic Press, 1983.

Sterba, Richard F. *Reminiscences of a Viennese Psychoanalyst.* Detroit: Wayne State University Press, 1982.

Stewart, Walter A. *Psychoanalysis: The First Ten Years 1888–1898.* New York: Macmillan, 1967.

Stone, Leo. *The Psychoanalytic Situation: An Examination of Its Development and Essential Nature.* New York: International Universities Press, 1961.

Strachey, James. "The Nature of the Therapeutic Action of Psycho-Analysis." *IJP* 15 (1934): 127–159.

——— "Notes on Some Technical Terms Whose Translation Calls for Comment." In *SE*, vol. 1.

Sulloway, Frank J. *Freud, Biologist of the Mind: Beyond the Psychoanalytic Legend.* New York: Basic Books, 1979.

——— "Freud and Biology: The Hidden Legacy." In *The Problematic Science: Psychology in Nineteenth-Century Thought,* edited by William R. Woodward and Mitchell G. Ash. New York: Praeger, 1982.

——— "Reassessing Freud's Case Histories: The Social Construction of Psychoanalysis." *ISIS* 82 (1991): 245–275.

Swales, Peter J. "Freud, Fliess, and Fratricide: The Role of Fliess in Freud's Conception of Paranoia." Privately printed, 1982.

——— "Freud, Martha Bernays, and the Language of Flowers." Privately printed, 1983.

——— "Freud, Krafft-Ebing, and the Witches: The Role of Krafft-Ebing in Freud's Flight into Fantasy." Privately printed, 1983.

——— "Freud, His Teacher, and the Birth of Psychoanalysis." In *Freud Appraisals and Reappraisals: Contributions to Freud Studies,* edited by Paul E. Stepansky, vol. 1. Hillsdale, N. J.: Analytic Press, 1986.

——— "Freud, Katharina, and the First 'Wild Analysis.'" In *Freud Appraisals and Reappraisals: Contributions to Freud Studies,* edited by Paul E. Stepansky, vol. 3. Hillsdale, N. J.: Analytic Press, 1988.

Taylor, Eugene. *William James on Exceptional Mental States: The 1896 Lowell Lectures.* New York: Charles Scribner's Sons, 1983.

Ticho, Ernst A. "The Influence of the German-Language Culture on Freud's Thought." *IJP* 67 (1986): 227–234.

Timms, Edward. "Freud's Library and His Private Reading." In *Freud in Exile: Psychoanalysis and Its Vicissitudes,* edited by Edward Timms and Naomi Segal. New Haven, Conn.: Yale University Press, 1988.

Timpanaro, Sebastiano. *The Freudian Slip: Psychoanalysis and Textual Criticism.* Translated by Kate Soper. London: Verso, 1985.

Toews, John E. "Historicizing Psychoanalysis: Freud in His Time and for Our Time." *Journal of Modern History* 63 (1991): 504–545.

Toulmin, Stephen, and David E. Leary. "The Cult of Empiricism in Psychology and Beyond." In *A Century of Psychology as Science,* edited by Sigmund Koch and David E. Leary. New York: McGraw-Hill, 1985.

Trosman, Harry, and Roger Dennis Simmons. "The Freud Library." *JAPA* 21 (1973): 646–687.

Turner, Frank Miller. *Between Science and Religion: The Reaction to Scientific Naturalism in Late Victorian England.* New Haven: Yale University Press, 1984.

Tyson, Robert L. "Countertransference Evolution in Theory and Practice." *JAPA* 34 (1986): 251–274.

Veith, Ilza. *Hysteria: The History of a Disease.* Chicago: University of Chicago Press, 1965.

Vermorel, Madelaine, and Henri Vermorel. "Was Freud a Romantic?" *IRP* 13 (1986): 15–37.

Vogel, L. Z. "The Case of Elise Gomperz." *American Journal of Psychoanalysis* 46 (1986): 230–238.

Wanner, Oskar. "Die Moser vom 'Charlottenfels.'" *Schweizer Archiv für Neurologie, Neurochirurgie und Psychiatrie* 131 (1982): 55–68.

Weiss, Stanley J. "Reflections and Speculations on the Psychoanalysis of the Rat Man." In *Freud and His Patients,* edited by Mark Kanzer and Jules Glenn. New York: Jason Aronson, 1980.

Whyte, L. L. *The Unconscious Before Freud.* New York: Basic Books, 1960

Widlocher, Daniel. "L'hysterie dépossédée." *Nouvelle revue de psychanalyse* 17 (1978): 73–87.

Wiener, Philip P. *Evolution and the Founders of Pragmatism.* Cambridge, Mass.: Harvard University Press, 1949.

Wild, John. *The Radical Empiricism of William James.* Garden City, N.Y.: Doubleday, 1969.

Williams, J. P. "Psychical Research and Psychiatry in Late Victorian Britain: Trance as Ecstasy or Trance as Insanity." In *The Anatomy of Madness: Essays in the History of Psychiatry.* Vol. 1, *People and Ideas,* edited by W. F. Bynum, Roy Porter, and Michael Shepherd. London: Tavistock Publications, 1985.

Wilshire, Bruce. *William James and Phenomenology: A Study of "The Principles of Psychology."* Bloomington, Ind.: Indiana University Press, 1968.

Wisdom, J. O. "What is Left of Psychoanalytic Theory?" *IRP* 11 (1984): 313–326.

Wittels, Fritz. *Sigmund Freud: His Personality, His Teaching, and His School.* Translated by Eden Paul and Ceder Paul. London: Allen and Unwin, 1924.

Wolfenstein, Eugene Victor. "A Man Who Knows Not Where to Have It: Habermas, Grünbaum and the Epistemological Status of Psychoanalysis." *IRP* 17 (1990): 23–45.

Wollheim, Richard. *Sigmund Freud.* New York: Viking Press, 1971. Reprint. Cambridge: Cambridge University Press, 1990.

—— "The Mind and the Mind's Image of Itself." In *On Art and the Mind: Essays and Lectures,* by Richard Wollheim. London: Allen Lane, 1973.

—— ed. *Freud: A Collection of Critical Essays.* Garden City, N.Y.: Doubleday, 1974.

Wollheim, Richard, and James Hopkins, eds. *Philosophical Essays on Freud.* Cambridge: Cambridge University Press, 1982.

Woodward, William. "Introduction." In *The Works of William James: Essays in Psychology.*

Wortis, Joseph. *Fragments of an Analysis with Freud.* New York: Simon and Schuster, 1954.

Yazmajian, Richard V. "Biological Aspects of Infantile Sexuality and the Latency Period." *The Psychoanalytic Quarterly* 36 (1967): 203–229.

Young-Bruehl, Elisabeth. *Anna Freud: A Biography.* New York: Summit Books, 1988.

Young, Robert M. *Mind, Brain and Adaptation in the Nineteenth Century: Cerebral Localization and Its Biological Context from Gall to Ferrier.* Oxford: Clarendon Press, 1970.

———— *Darwin's Metaphor: Nature's Place in Victorian Culture.* New York: Cambridge University Press, 1985.

———— "Freud: Scientist and/or Humanist." *Free Associations* 6 (1986): 7–35.

Zanuso, Billa. *The Young Freud: The Origins of Psychoanalysis in the Late Nineteenth-Century Viennese Culture.* Oxford: Basil Blackwell, 1986.

Zetzel, Elizabeth R. "1965: Additional Notes upon a Case of Obsessional Neurosis: Freud 1909." *IJP* 47 (1966): 123–129.

———— *The Capacity for Emotional Growth.* London: Hogarth Press; New York: International Universities Press, 1972.

Zilboorg, Gregory, in collaboration with George W. Henry. *A History of Medical Psychology.* New York: Norton, 1941.

Index

Index

Index

Myers, Frederick W. H., 13, 14; "The Subliminal Consciousness," 6, 11

Narcissism, 95, 96, 99, 108
Neurasthenia, 36, 39, 41, 44, 78, 100
Neurology, 17–18, 37, 100
Neuropathology, 45
Neurosis, 36, 112; anxiety, 36, 39, 40–42, 43–44, 50–52, 78, 81, 82, 117, 131, 133, 164; choice of, 60, 61; defense, 34, 78, 81, 86, 134, 166; infantile, 103; nuclear complex in, 86–87, 103; obsessional, 50, 78, 87–94, 103, 108, 150; and sexuality, 37, 144; transference, 157–158, 159
Nietzsche, Friedrich, 66
"Note on the Unconscious in Psycho-Analysis" (Freud), 13–15

Oedipus complex, 83–84, 94, 103, 127, 158, 166–167
Oedipus Rex (Sophocles), 83–84
"On Narcissism: An Introduction" (Freud), 108

Pain, 63, 128, 132, 133, 134, 142; and hysteria, 31–32, 35, 45, 129, 164
Paneth, Josef, 140
Pankejeff, Anna, 100
Pankejeff, Sergei (Wolf Man), 99–108, 166, 167
Pappenheim, Bertha (Anna O.), 22–27, 29, 31, 110, 112, 161, 164
Paranoia, 59, 60, 86, 95, 102; and projection, 60–61
Parapsychology, 14
Parents, death of, 83–84
Patient-doctor relationship, 110–117, 124–125, 161
Personality: division of, 6, 8–11, 159
Perversions, 85, 96
Philosophy, 13, 65–66, 163, 164, 165, 167, 168
Phobias, 39, 53, 84; animal, 103, 104–108
Physiology, 22, 38, 145, 164, 165, 167
Presentations: word vs. thing, 16–17, 18
Pressure technique, 113, 115, 116, 118, 123

"Project for a Scientific Psychology" (Freud), 18, 167
Projection, 60–61, 159
Psyche: and soma, 22–36, 164
Psychoanalysis, 46, 53, 61, 100, 102, 103, 112, 118, 151–152, 167–168; as archeology, 74, 78, 92, 104, 165–166; and concept of the unconscious, 1, 13, 20; as a discipline, 1–2, 167, 168; history of, 1, 3; principles of, 87, 149, 153, 159, 162; and self-analysis, 161. *See also* Freud, Sigmund: self-analysis of; Transference
"Psycho-Analytic Notes on an Autobiographical Account of a Case of Paranoia" (Freud), 60
"The Psychogenesis of a Case of Homosexuality in a Woman" (Freud), 125
Psychology, 2, 5, 12, 13, 21, 38, 135, 148, 164; and philosophy, 21, 65, 163
Psychopathology, 60
The Psychopathology of Everyday Life (Freud), 73, 118, 144
Psychosexuality, 2, 42, 44, 45, 164, 166

Rat Man. *See* Lanzer, Dr. Ernst
"Remembering, Repeating and Working-Through" (Freud), 69
Repression, 17, 18, 114–115, 119; and censorship, 20
Resistance, 152, 154, 156, 160, 161
Roff, Mary. *See* Vennum, Lurancy
Rosanes, Ignaz, 132, 133

Sadism, 51, 85–86
Sanatorium Bellevue (Kreuzlingen), 23
Schizophrenia, 15–16
Schreber, Daniel Gottlob Moritz, 58
Schreber, Daniel Paul, 58–63, 95, 96, 108, 165
Science, 1, 13, 66, 168
"Screen Memories" (Freud), 66
Sexuality, 38–39, 109, 110–111, 164; components of, 84–85; and hostility, 111–112, 125; infantile, 38, 45–46, 51–52, 79, 82, 83–84, 92, 93, 96, 103, 104, 106, 117, 158; and neuroses, 37, 51, 81, 101, 131. *See also* Psychosexuality
"Sexuality in the Aetiology of the Neuroses" (Freud), 36